Posttraumatic Stress Disorder
Acute and Long-Term Responses
to Trauma and Disaster

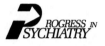

David Spiegel, M.D.
Series Editor

Posttraumatic Stress Disorder

Acute and Long-Term Responses to Trauma and Disaster

Edited by Carol S. Fullerton, Ph.D., and Robert J. Ursano, M.D.

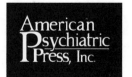

Washington, DC
London, England

Copyright © 1997 American Psychiatric Press, Inc.

ALL RIGHTS RESERVED

Manufactured in the United States of America on acid-free paper

First Edition   00   99   98   97   4   3   2   1

American Psychiatric Press, Inc.
1400 K Street, N.W., Washington, DC   20005

Library of Congress Cataloging-in-Publication Data
Posttraumatic stress disorder : acute and long-term responses to trauma and
    disaster / edited by Carol S. Fullerton and Robert J. Ursano. — 1st ed.
        p. cm. — (Progress in psychiatry series ; #51)
    Includes bibliographical references and index.
    ISBN 0-88048-751-8 (cloth : alk. paper)
    1. Post-traumatic stress disorder. I. Fullerton, Carol S.
II. Ursano, Robert J., 1947-   . III. Series.
    [DNLM: 1. Stress Disorders, Post-Traumatic. 2. Stress,
Psychological—complications. W1 PR6781L no. 51 1997 / WM 170 P8572
1997]
RC552.P67P666 1997
616.85'21—dc20
DNLM/DLC
for Library of Congress   96-24027
                                                                                                          CIP

British Library Cataloguing in Publication Data
A CIP record is available from the British Library.

Contents

Contributors

Tim A. Bullman, M.A.
Statistician, Environmental Epidemiology Service, Department of Veterans Affairs, Washington, DC

Dennis S. Charney, M.D.
Chief, Psychiatry Service, Clinical Neurosciences Division, National Center for Posttraumatic Stress Disorder, West Haven VA Medical Center, New Haven, Connecticut; Professor of Psychiatry, Department of Psychiatry, Yale University School of Medicine, New Haven, Connecticut

Catherine Classen, Ph.D.
Social Science Research Associate, Psychosocial Treatment Laboratory, Department of Psychiatry and Behavioral Sciences, Stanford University School of Medicine, Stanford, California

Raina E. Eberly, Ph.D.
Staff Psychologist, Department of Psychology, Department of Veterans Affairs Medical Center, Minneapolis, Minnesota; Clinical Associate Professor of Psychology, Department of Psychology, University of Minnesota, Minneapolis, Minnesota

Brian E. Engdahl, Ph.D.
Staff Psychologist, Department of Psychology, Department of Veterans Affairs Medical Center, Minneapolis, Minnesota; Clinical Associate Professor of Psychology, Department of Psychology, University of Minnesota, Minneapolis, Minnesota

Alan Fontana, Ph.D.
Associate Director, PTSD Program, Northeast Program Evaluation Center, West Haven VA Medical Center, New Haven, Connecticut; Senior Research Scientist, Department of Psychiatry, Yale University School of Medicine, New Haven, Connecticut

Linda Frisman, Ph.D.
Associate Director, Health Care for Homeless Veterans, Northeast Program Evaluation Center, West Haven VA Medical Center, New Haven, Connecticut; Associate Research Scientist, Department of Psychiatry, Yale University School of Medicine, New Haven, Connecticut

Carol S. Fullerton, Ph.D.
Associate Professor (Research), Department of Psychiatry, Uniformed Services University of the Health Sciences, F. Edward Hébert School of Medicine, Bethesda, Maryland

Kenneth J. Hoffman, M.D., M.P.H.
Assistant Professor, Departments of Preventive Medicine and Psychiatry, Uniformed Services University of the Health Sciences, F. Edward Hébert School of Medicine, Bethesda, Maryland

Han K. Kang, Dr.P.H.
Director, Environmental Epidemiology Service, Department of Veterans Affairs, Washington, DC

Elie G. Karam, M.D.
Professor, Department of Psychiatry, Faculty of Medicine, Psychiatry and Psychology Clinical and Research Program, American University of Beirut, Lebanon

Cheryl Koopman, Ph.D.
Senior Research Associate, Psychosocial Treatment Laboratory, Department of Psychiatry and Behavioral Sciences, Stanford University School of Medicine, Stanford, California

Catherine Leda, M.S.N., M.P.H.
Associate Director, Domiciliary Care for Homeless Veterans, Compensated Work, Therapy/Therapeutic Residency Programs, Northeast Program Evaluation Center, West Haven VA Medical Center, New Haven, Connecticut; Associate Research Scientist, Department of Psychiatry, Yale University School of Medicine, New Haven, Connecticut

James E. McCarroll, Ph.D.
Research Psychologist, Department of Military Psychiatry, Walter Reed Army Institute of Research, Washington, DC

William F. Page, Ph.D.
Senior Program Officer, Medical Follow-Up Agency, Institute of Medicine, National Academy of Sciences, Washington, DC

Robert Rosenheck, M.D.
Director, Northeast Program Evaluation Center, Deputy Chief, Resources and Program Development, Evaluation Division, National Center for Posttraumatic Stress Disorder, West Haven VA Medical Center, New Haven, Connecticut; Clinical Professor, Department of Psychiatry, Yale University, New Haven, Connecticut

Jane E. Sasaki, M.D.
Assistant Professor, Department of Psychiatry, Uniformed Services University of the Health Sciences, F. Edward Hébert School of Medicine, Bethesda, Maryland

Arieh Y. Shalev, M.D.
Associate Professor of Psychiatry, Department of Psychiatry, Director, Center for Traumatic Stress, Hadassah University Hospital, Jerusalem, Israel

Jon A. Shaw, M.D.
Professor and Director, Division of Child and Adolescent Psychiatry, University of Miami School of Medicine, Miami, Florida

Steven M. Southwick, M.D.
Director, Posttraumatic Stress Disorder Program, Clinical Neurosciences Division, National Center for Posttraumatic Stress Disorder, West Haven VA Medical Center, New Haven, Connecticut; Associate Professor of Psychiatry, Department of Psychiatry, Yale University School of Medicine, New Haven, Connecticut

David Spiegel, M.D.
Professor of Psychiatry and Behavioral Sciences, Department of Psychiatry and Behavioral Sciences, Stanford University School of Medicine, Stanford, California

Robert J. Ursano, M.D.
Professor and Chairman, Department of Psychiatry, Uniformed Services University of the Health Sciences, F. Edward Hébert School of Medicine, Bethesda, Maryland

Lars Weisæth, M.D., Ph.D.
Professor and Head, Division of Disaster Psychiatry, Medical Faculty, University of Oslo, Oslo, Norway; Head, Department of Psychiatry, Joint Norwegian Armed Forces Medical Services, Norway

Rachel Yehuda, Ph.D.
Assistant Professor of Psychiatry, Director, Traumatic Stress Studies Program, Psychiatry Department, Mt. Sinai School of Medicine, New York, New York; Director, PTSD Program, Department of Psychiatry, Bronx VA Medical Center, Bronx, New York

Introduction to the Progress in Psychiatry Series

The Progress in Psychiatry Series is designed to capture in print the excitement that comes from assembling a diverse group of experts from various locations to examine in detail the newest information about a developing aspect of psychiatry. This series emerged as a collaboration between the American Psychiatric Association's (APA) Scientific Program Committee and the American Psychiatric Press, Inc. Great interest is generated by a number of the symposia presented each year at the APA annual meeting, and we realized that much of the information presented there, carefully assembled by people who are deeply immersed in a given area, would unfortunately not appear together in print. The symposia sessions at the annual meetings provide an unusual opportunity for experts who otherwise might not meet on the same platform to share their diverse viewpoints for 3 hours. Some new themes are repeatedly reinforced and gain credence, whereas in other instances disagreements emerge, enabling the audience and now the reader to reach informed decisions about new directions in the field. The Progress in Psychiatry Series allows us to publish and capture some of the best of the symposia and thus provide an in-depth treatment of specific areas that might not otherwise be presented in broader review formats.

Psychiatry is, by nature, an interface discipline, combining the study of mind and brain, of individual and social environments, and of the humane and the scientific. Therefore, progress in the field is rarely linear—it often comes from unexpected sources. Furthermore, new developments emerge from an array of viewpoints that do not necessarily provide immediate agreement but rather expert examination of the issues. We intend to present innovative ideas and data that will enable you, the reader, to participate in this process.

We believe the Progress in Psychiatry Series will provide you with an opportunity to review timely, new information in specific fields of interest as they are developing. We hope you find that the excitement of the presentations is captured in the written word and that this book proves to be informative and enjoyable reading.

David Spiegel, M.D.
Series Editor
Progress in Psychiatry Series

Part I

Introduction

Chapter 1

The Other Side of Chaos: Understanding the Patterns of Posttraumatic Responses

Carol S. Fullerton, Ph.D., and Robert J. Ursano, M.D.

Trauma is always a catalyst for change and adjustment. Over time, most people exposed to trauma will do well; some, however, do not. A complex interaction of environment, biology, and mind determines which individuals develop posttraumatic psychiatric disease. Studies suggest that acute posttraumatic responses predict the development of chronic posttraumatic stress disorder (PTSD) (e.g., Baum 1987; Breslau and Davis 1987; Breslau et al. 1991; Green et al. 1990a, 1990b; Shore et al. 1989), although the point at which acute stress reactions become of clinical concern remains unclear (Green and Lindy 1994). Psychiatrists assume that early detection and intervention will prevent the development of chronic PTSD; systematic empirical research concerning this clinical impression, however, is lacking (S. D. Solomon et al. 1992).

Trauma and disasters throw lives into chaos and fill people with terror of the unexpected and fear of loss, injury, and death. The human chaos of trauma, however, is not random. Rather, posttraumatic stress responses frequently have a predictable structure and time course (Ursano et al. 1994a). Several empirical studies have examined responses to trauma, war, and disaster events (e.g., Breslau et al. 1991; Green and Lindy 1993, 1994; Norris and Kaniasty 1992; Steinglass and Gerrity 1990; Ursano and Fullerton 1990; Ursano et al. 1992a; Weisæth and Eitinger 1993).

The past decade has seen dramatic increases in psychiatry's understanding of biopsychosocial responses to trauma and disasters (see Davidson and Foa 1993; Green and Lindy 1994; Ursano et al. 1994b;

Wilson and Raphael 1993). For most individuals, posttraumatic psychiatric symptoms are transitory. For some, however, the effects of a disaster linger long after the traumatic event has passed, recalled in memory by new experiences that remind the person of the past traumatic event (Holloway and Ursano 1984; Lifton 1993; Ursano and Fullerton 1990; Ursano et al. 1994a; Weisæth 1989a, 1989b).

This book presents state-of-the-art knowledge regarding the effects of trauma and disasters on psychiatric health; it emphasizes current and developing advances and directions. This book follows the arrival of DSM-IV (American Psychiatric Association 1994) and the new diagnostic category *Acute Stress Disorder* (ASD). This additional diagnosis emphasizes the breadth of posttraumatic stress symptoms and disorders and the importance of distinguishing acute and long-term responses to traumatic events. Practitioners must consider the full range of disorders to develop interventions appropriate to posttraumatic distress and illness.

This book takes a broad integrative approach to the investigation of posttraumatic stress disorders. Its chapters demonstrate the interface of emotions, cognitions, biology, and the environment. This book brings together clinical, observational reports and empirical studies; these findings convey their own stories and make them useful for clinicians, researchers, and policy makers. This volume highlights practical implications and areas that require further study.

This work makes a unique contribution in its integration of disaster, war, and other trauma studies. The format and content of this book highlight the commonalties as well as the unique factors among traumatic events. Identifying the characteristic patterns of posttraumatic responses across traumatic events is important to improve psychiatry's understanding of etiological processes underlying the effects of trauma. The authors in this volume consider posttraumatic responses across individual, group, family, and community perspectives and from the vantage point of developmental systems from childhood to older adult life. Each level of description leads to more in-depth understanding, with implications for research, service provision, and policy and planning. This volume also identifies psychosocial contexts, as well as culture, as important moderating processes. We hope this book is a valuable and creative stimulus to psychiatry's knowledge of the human chaos that occurs when individuals and communities are exposed to horrific and life-threatening situations.

BACKGROUND

The Thousand-Mile Stare and Other War Neuroses

The study of emotional reactions to disasters began with observations of the oldest nonnatural disaster: war. During the Civil War, trauma casualties were thought to be suffering from "nostalgia." Large numbers of soldiers reported symptoms of generalized weakness, heart palpitations, and chest pain. Physicians used terms such as "soldier's heart," "irritable heart," and "effort syndrome" to describe what they thought were biological conditions resulting from physical stress experienced by soldiers. Physicians observed clustering of trauma-related symptoms in the early wars of this century. Later, in World War II, physicians commonly used terms such as "shell shock," "battle fatigue," and "war neuroses" to describe soldiers experiencing fatigue, exhaustion, and anxiety; the "thousand-mile stare" described the exhausted foot soldier on the verge of collapse.

From these observations, the study of other disasters began. Between the world wars, individuals in railway accidents sought relief from symptoms of chronic pain, anxiety, and invalidism. Some physicians thought these symptoms were caused by neurologic injury (e.g., "railway spine"), whereas others believed the symptoms to be fabrications ("compensation neurosis").

The development of standardized diagnostic instruments such as the Structured Clinical Interview (SCID) for DSM-III-R (American Psychiatric Association 1987) and the Diagnostic Interview Schedule (DIS) (Robins et al. 1981) have facilitated controlled systematic research on PTSD in a wide range of trauma and disaster populations. Generalization and long-term follow-up, however, remain uneven because of diverse methodologies and conceptualizations. The nature of disaster events—the unpredictable onset and severity of disasters, the lack of baseline data, the difficulty of obtaining control groups, and high rates of attrition—exacerbates these difficulties. Despite these methodological problems and limitations, psychiatrists are learning a great deal about the psychiatric effects of trauma by examining the broad range of traumatic events and disasters.

Positive Aspects of Trauma and its Aftermath

For some people, trauma and loss facilitate a move toward health (Card 1983; Lifton 1993; Sledge et al. 1980; Ursano 1981). A traumatic experience can become the center around which an individual reorganizes a previously disorganized life, reorienting values and goals (Ursano 1981, 1987). Traumatic events appear to function as psychic organizers—psychic glue that links affects, cognitions, and behaviors that are later expressed after symbolic, environmental, or biological stimuli (Holloway and Ursano 1984).

For example, although many survivors of a 1974 tornado in Xenia, Ohio, experienced psychological distress, the majority described positive outcomes: learning that they could handle crises effectively and feeling that they were better off for having met this type of challenge (Quarentelli 1985; Taylor 1977). Sledge et al. (1980) found that approximately one-third of U.S. Air Force Vietnam-era prisoners of war (POWs) reported that they benefited from their POW experiences; moreover, these POWs tended to be the ones who had suffered the most traumatic experiences.

Posttraumatic Stress Disorder

With the introduction of PTSD as a diagnosis in DSM-III (American Psychiatric Association 1980), research on the psychiatric effects of trauma and disaster increased dramatically. The description of PTSD was refined in DSM-III-R, which defined the stressor criterion operationally and provided information about symptoms in a broader range of populations, including traumatized children. DSM-IV changed the criteria for PTSD to emphasize exposure to life threat as the stressor and to move physiologic symptoms related to reminders of the disaster event into the remembering criteria (Criteria B) rather than the arousal criteria (Criteria D).

With regard to trauma involving a loved one, the diagnostic criteria also vary slightly between DSM-III-R and DSM-IV, although the intent is the same. DSM-III-R specified that stressors meeting PTSD diagnostic criteria included ". . . a serious threat or harm to one's children, spouse, or other close relatives and friends" (p. 250). DSM-IV specifies ". . . events experienced by others that are learned about include, but are not limited to, violent personal assault, serious accident, or serious injury experienced by a family member or a close friend; learning about the sudden unexpected death of a family member or close friend . . . " (p. 424). According to DSM-IV, the higher the intensity of the stressor and the closer the physical proximity to the stressor, the greater the risk for developing PTSD.

Acute Stress Disorder

Research on acute posttraumatic stress responses has been limited by the absence of a specific diagnostic category for early posttraumatic stress symptoms. Importantly, estimates of the prevalence of PTSDs have not included what is perhaps the largest group of people exposed to trauma: those with symptoms that last only several days to weeks posttrauma. ASD, introduced in DSM-IV, is characterized by posttraumatic stress symptoms lasting at least 2 days but not longer that 1 month posttrauma.

Other Psychiatric Disorders Associated with Traumatic Stress

PTSD and ASD are not the only psychiatric disorders associated with disasters. In fact, they may not even be the most common. PTSD, major depression, substance abuse, generalized anxiety disorder, and adjustment disorder have all been noted following disasters and trauma (Rundell et al. 1989). In addition, psychological reactions to physical injury and illness, as well as psychological resiliency, are important postdisaster responses.

EPIDEMIOLOGY OF TRAUMATIC EVENTS AND POSTTRAUMATIC STRESS DISORDERS

A large proportion of the population of the United States is affected by disasters (Federal Emergency Management Agency 1984; Rubin and Nahavandian 1987). Norris (1988) estimated that 6% to 7% of the United States population is exposed to a disaster or trauma each year, ranging from motor vehicle accidents and crime to hurricanes and tornadoes. Disasters and trauma effect psychological and physical health and are extremely costly, as well as traumatic. Hundreds of thousands of people—victims, their relatives, their friends, disaster workers, and witnesses—are affected every year.

The health and financial costs of disasters are enormous. Between 1965 and 1985, 31 states experienced five or more presidentially declared disasters. Direct federal assistance from the Federal Emergency Management Agency (FEMA) totaled more than $6 billion from 1965 to 1985. In 1989 the American Red Cross spent $14 million for the victims of Hurricane Hugo and $19.5 million for the victims of the Loma Prieta earthquake in California. More recently, the estimated cost of the 1994 Los Angeles earthquake is now expected to exceed $10 billion. The effects of such events extend well beyond the direct victims to include families, communities, and those who try to help: All become part of the trauma and disaster community.

Recognizing the growth in psychiatry's knowledge regarding responses to disaster, the widespread nature of disasters in the modern world, and the importance of psychiatric care to disaster victims, the American Psychiatric Association established first a task force in 1991 and in 1993 established the Committee on Psychiatric Dimensions of Disaster. This committee and its local district branches focuses on developing direct care models, consulting to disaster communities, and educating psychiatrists in the skills and knowledge of disaster psychiatry.

POSTTRAUMATIC STRESS DISORDERS

Posttraumatic Stress Disorder

PTSD has been widely studied—initially in Vietnam veterans and subsequently in natural and nonnatural disasters other than war, as well as criminal violence (Kilpatrick and Resnick 1993; McFarlane 1988b; Shore et al. 1986, 1989; Smith and North 1993; Steinglass and Gerrity 1990). The study of Vietnam veterans contributed greatly to psychiatry's understanding of PTSD (Davidson and Fairbank 1992; Kulka et al. 1990, 1991). Researchers have now examined posttraumatic psychiatric responses in survivors of airplane crashes, volcanic eruptions, tornadoes, floods, criminal victimization, and other disasters. Other studies have examined PTSD-equivalent disorders resulting from the Coconut Grove fire (Adler 1943), the Buffalo Creek dam collapse (Titchener and Kapp 1976), and other disasters. Most studies have found that the best predictor of PTSD is the degree of exposure to the disaster. The greatest risk of PTSD is in persons exposed to life threat and, perhaps, in those exposed to terror, horror, and the grotesque (Lima et al. 1987; Parker 1977; Ursano and McCarroll 1990; Ursano et al. 1995). Psychiatrists know much less about acute PTSD than chronic PTSD (Ursano et al. 1992b, Ursano 1995).

The Epidemiological Catchment Area (ECA) study found prevalence rates of PTSD in the general population of 1.0% to 2.6% (Davidson and Fairbank 1992; Helzer et al. 1987). Helzer et al. (1987) found a 1% lifetime prevalence of PTSD in adults from the St. Louis ECA site. Incidence rates in populations at risk (those exposed to extreme stressors) ranged from 3.3% to 6.3%. Much higher rates of PTSD have been found subsequently by other investigators studying exposed groups. In the North Carolina ECA survey site, Davidson and Fairbank (1992) found a 1.3% lifetime prevalence among adults in the Piedmont region.

In a random sample of young adults from a health maintenance organization in Detroit, Breslau et al. (1991) estimated that the lifetime prevalence of exposure to traumatic events was 39.1%; these investigators found a 9% lifetime prevalence of PTSD. Of those who had experienced a traumatic event, 23.6% developed PTSD, and 57% of this group experienced symptoms for 1 year or more. In this population—nearly all of whom reported chronic rather than acute PTSD—risk factors for PTSD following a traumatic event included early separation from parents, neuroticism, preexisting anxiety or depression, and family history of anxiety.

In one of the earliest epidemiological studies of combat veterans, using the ECA data, Helzer et al. (1987) found the incidence of PTSD in combat veterans to be 6.3%. In a large study of Israeli soldiers ($N = 3,553$) with acute combat stress reaction during the 1982 Lebanon War, Z. Solomon and Benbenishty (1986) found chronic PTSD rates of 56% 2 years after combat exposure.

The National Vietnam Veterans Readjustment Study (NVVRS) (Kulka et al. 1990, 1991) is the most extensive epidemiological study to date of the long-term psychiatric effects of combat. The prevalence of PTSD in Vietnam veterans up to 19 years after war was 15% (Kulka et al. 1990). Preliminary studies of Persian Gulf war veterans during the first year after return indicated that approximately 9% of veterans exhibited PTSD (Rosenheck et al. 1992).

The incidence of psychiatric disorders after combat is positively associated with the degree of war trauma experienced, witnessing/ participating in atrocities, and being wounded (Kulka et al. 1990, 1991; Sutker et al. 1991; Ursano et al. 1981). In addition to combat severity, other factors contribute to the risk of psychiatric disorder following combat. The NVVRS study, as well as most other studies of clinical populations of PTSD, found high comorbid rates of depression, anxiety disorders, and substance abuse in veterans with chronic PTSD.

The ECA study of Vietnam veterans documented a higher rate of PTSD in wounded Vietnam veterans (Helzer et al. 1987), and the NVVRS study noted similar findings (Kulka et al. 1990, 1991). Greater exposure to combat in Vietnam also was significantly related to higher rates of PTSD, depression, and alcohol abuse (Kulka et al. 1990).

In an interesting study, Goldberg et al. (1987) studied monozygotic twins who were discordant for service in Vietnam. Of the twins who had served in Vietnam, 16.8% had PTSD; in contrast, only 5% of the twins who had not served had PTSD. The prevalence of PTSD in the twins exposed to high levels of combat in Vietnam was nine times higher than that in their noncombat siblings.

Acute Stress Disorder

A diagnostic category for acute responses to trauma and disaster events was curiously absent from DSM-III and DSM-III-R. DSM-IV acknowledges a broader spectrum of responses to traumatic events, with the new diagnosis of ASD. ASD symptoms occur within 4 weeks of a traumatic event and last between 2 days and 4 weeks.

Because this is a new diagnosis, no specific studies are available on its course or outcome (Spiegel and Cardeña 1993). Recent studies of war suggest that sustained combat-related ASD predicts an adverse outcome (Z. Solomon and Mikulincer 1987) and is associated with increased rates of somatic complaints (Z. Solomon et al. 1987). Numerous studies also document that acute symptoms of intrusion, avoidance, and dissociation (Cardeña and Spiegel 1993)—part of the symptom complex of ASD—predict the development of later psychiatric disorders, particularly PTSD (Perry et al. 1992; Smith and North 1993; van der Kolk and van der Hart 1989; Weisæth 1989a, 1989b, 1994).

Depression, Substance Abuse, Anxiety, and Adjustment Disorders

Researchers have less often studied major depression, generalized anxiety disorder, and substance abuse, but available data suggest higher rates of these disorders in most disaster populations (Kulka et al. 1990; Rundell et al. 1989; Shore et al. 1986, 1989; Smith et al. 1989). Depression and substance abuse also are common comorbid disorders in studies of PTSD, most of which are studies of chronic PTSD (see Davidson and Fairbank 1992; Keane and Wolfe 1990; Rundell et al. 1989; Smith and North 1993; Smith et al. 1986). In survivors of a plane crash, for example, PTSD co-occurred with depression or generalized anxiety disorder four times more frequently than it did by itself (Smith et al. 1989).

Other

Physicians often overlook psychiatric disorders attributable to head injury and metabolic disturbances following incidents involving crush injuries and burns. Diagnoses of psychological factors affecting physical disease and PTSD are frequent in injured persons who must deal with the stress of their injury, the loss of family members, and the absence of resources and social supports with which to plan recovery. Similarly, investigators have rarely examined the issues of potential family violence (spouse abuse and child abuse) in stressed families following major disasters and increased behavioral disorders in children; psychiatrists often neglect these factors in clinical work following traumatic events.

THE IMPACT OF TRAUMA OVER TIME

Few studies have addressed psychiatric responses to trauma over time, yet acute and long-term responses appear to be quite different clinically and may be extremely important to distinguish. Smith and North (1993) found systematic longitudinal research on PTSD in particular to be lacking, although there are several notable exceptions. Green et al. (1989) studied survivors of the Buffalo Creek disaster and found that the rates of PTSD were 44% at 18 to 26 months and 28% at 14 years after the disaster. The rates of PTSD in flood survivors examined by Steinglass and Gerrity (1990) were 14.5% at 4 months and 4.5% at 16 months after the disaster. Steinglass and Gerrity (1990) found PTSD in 21% of one community's population 16 months after a tornado. McFarlane (1986, 1988a) studied disaster workers following a bush fire and also showed long-term psychiatric morbidity using the General Health Questionnaire (GHQ) (Goldberg 1972).

Kilpatrick et al. (1987) found PTSD prevalence rates of 7.5% in women (N = 391) who were criminally assaulted (an average of 15 years after the trauma). In another community sample (N = 214), Kilpatrick et al. (1989, 1990) found that 29% of adult family survivors of criminal homicide experienced PTSD at some point after the murder; this proportion dropped to 7% at the time of inquiry (time not specified). In a sample of alcohol-related vehicular homicide survivors, 34.1% reported PTSD at some point after the accident, and 2.2% reported PTSD at the time of inquiry. These findings suggest that in these community samples, only a small proportion of persons with acute PTSD develop chronic PTSD (see Kilpatrick and Resnick 1993 for a review of empirical studies of criminal assault). Similarly, Ursano et al. (1995) found significant PTSD in disaster workers shortly after exposure to human remains, but recovery tended to occur by 1 year later.

Issues involving acute versus chronic responses to trauma and disaster are manifold for all posttraumatic stress responses, not just PTSD. Who is at risk of acute disorders? Who is at risk of chronic disorders? Who recovers? What are the predictors of long-term and short-term risk? Are they the same or different? How might the answers to these questions guide our interventions—such as the use of medications (antidepressants, hypnotics, antianxiety agents) and psychotherapy (debriefing, focus on the traumatic event, focus on disease sustaining factors)?

Investigators must be alert to which type of disorder (acute versus chronic) they are studying in any research program. Insufficient attention to the dimension of acute versus chronic illness has led to incomplete consideration of both ends of the spectrum with regard to the new diagnosis of ASD, depression (see Chapter 5), and the issues of family violence and substance abuse after major community disruptions such as the Persian Gulf War (see Chapter 6) or Hurricane Andrew (see Chapter 7).

CONCLUSIONS

Despite a large body of literature, there are substantial gaps in psychiatry's current understanding of responses to trauma and its outcomes, as well as methods to assist victims. In response to this need, this volume brings together clinical and research issues regarding acute and long-term posttraumatic responses. Respected national and international investigators and medical professionals, at the cutting edge of innovative methodologies, examine medical issues critical to research and practical treatment of trauma and disaster groups.

The chapters in this volume go beyond PTSD to examine other posttraumatic disorders and responses, the mechanisms of transmission of posttraumatic stress, and its effects on behavior and health in natural and nonnatural (including war) disasters and traumas. The authors pay particular attention to the array of psychiatric responses to trauma, including but not limited to PTSD, and the longitudinal unfolding of illness and recovery. By adopting both "oil-emersion" and "wide angle" views of traumatic responses, we hope to take the reader beyond the chaos of the effects of disasters toward the underlying structures and mechanisms of these events across time.

REFERENCES

Adler A: Neuropsychiatric complications in victims of Boston's Coconut Grove disaster. JAMA 123:1098–1101, 1943

American Psychiatric Association: Diagnosis and Statistical Manual of Mental Disorders, 3rd Edition. Washington, DC, American Psychiatric Association, 1980

American Psychiatric Association: Diagnosis and Statistical Manual of Mental Disorders, 3rd Edition, Revised. Washington, DC: American Psychiatric Association, 1987

American Psychiatric Association: Diagnostic and Statistical Manual of Mental Disorders, 4th Edition. Washington, DC, American Psychiatric Association, 1994

Baum A: Toxins, technology, and natural disasters, in Cataclysms, Crises, and Catastrophes: Psychology in Action. Edited by Vanden Bos GR, Bryant BD. Washington, DC, American Psychological Association, 1987, pp 5–54

Breslau N, Davis GC: Post-traumatic stress disorder: the etiologic specificity of wartime stressors. Am J Psychiatry 144:578–583, 1987

Breslau N, Davis GC, Andreski P, et al: Traumatic events and posttraumatic stress disorder in a urban population of young adults. Arch Gen Psychiatry 48:216–222, 1991

Card JJ: Lives after Vietnam. Lexington, MA, Lexington Books, 1983

Cardeña E, Spiegel D: Dissociative reactions of the San Francisco Bay area earthquake of 1989. Am J Psychiatry 150:474–478, 1993

Davidson JRT, Fairbank JA: The epidemiology of posttraumatic stress disorder, in Posttraumatic Stress Disorder: DSM-IV and Beyond. Edited by Davidson JRT, Foa EB. Washington, DC, American Psychiatric Press, 1992, pp 147–172

Davidson JRT, Foa EB (eds): Posttraumatic Stress Disorder: DSM-IV and Beyond. Washington, DC, American Psychiatric Press, 1993

Federal Emergency Management Agency (FEMA): Program Guide, Disaster Assistance Programs. Washington, DC, U.S. Government Printing Office, 1984

Goldberg DP: The detection of psychiatric illness by questionnaire. Maudsley Monograph 21. London, Oxford University Press, 1972

Goldberg J, True W, Eisen S, et al: The Vietnam Era Twin (VET) registry: ascertainment bias. Acta Genet Med Gemellol (Roma) 36:67–78, 1987

Green BL, Lindy JD: Identifying survivors at risk: trauma and stressors across events, in International Handbook of Traumatic Stress Syndromes. Edited by Wilson JP, Raphael B. New York, Plenum, 1993, pp 135–144

Green BL, Lindy JD: Post-traumatic stress disorder in victims of disasters. Psychiatr Clin North Am 17:301–309, 1994

Green BL, Lindy JD, Grace MC, et al: Multiple diagnosis in posttraumatic stress disorder: the role of war stressors. J Nerv Ment Dis 177: 329–335, 1989

Green BL, Grace MC, Lindy JD, et al: War stressor and symptom persistence in posttraumatic stress disorder. Journal of Anxiety Disorders 4:31–39, 1990a

Green BL, Lindy JD, Grace MC, et al: Buffalo Creek survivors in the second decade: stability of stress symptoms. Am J Orthopsychiatry 60:43–54, 1990b

Helzer JE, Robins LN, McEvoy L: Post-traumatic stress disorder in the general population. N Engl J Med 317:1630–1634, 1987

Holloway HC, Ursano RJ: The Vietnam veteran: memory, social context, and metaphor. Psychiatry 47:103–108, 1984

Keane TM, Wolfe J: Comorbidity in post-traumatic stress disorder: an analysis of community and clinical studies. Journal of Applied Social Psychology 20:1776–1788, 1990

Kilpatrick DG, Resnick HS: Posttraumatic stress disorder associated with exposure to criminal victimization in clinical and community populations, in Posttraumatic Stress Disorder: DSM-IV and Beyond. Edited by Davidson JRT, Foa EB. Washington, DC, American Psychiatric Press, 1993, pp 113–143

Kilpatrick DG, Saunders BE, Veronen LJ, et al: Criminal victimization: lifetime prevalence, reporting to police, and psychological impact. Crime and Delinquency 33:479–489, 1987

Kilpatrick DG, Resnick HS, Amick A: Family members of homicide victims: search for meaning and post-traumatic stress disorder. Paper presented at the 97th annual convention of the American Psychological Association, New Orleans, LA, August 1989

Kilpatrick DG, Amick A, Resnick HS: The impact of homicide on surviving family members. Final Report, National Institute of Justice, Grant No. 87-IJ-CX-0017, 1990

Kulka RA, Schlenger WE, Fairbank JA, et al: Trauma and the Vietnam War Generation. New York, Brunner/Mazel, 1990

Kulka RA, Schlenger WE, Fairbank JA, et al: Assessment of posttraumatic stress disorder in the community: prospects and pitfalls from recent studies of Vietnam veterans. Psychological Assesment: A Journal of Consulting and Clinical Psychology 3:547–560, 1991

Lifton RJ: The Protean Self: Human Resilience in an Age of Fragmentation. New York, Basic Books, 1993

Lima BR, Pai S, Santacruz H, et al: Screening for the psychological consequences of a major disaster in a developing country: Amero, Colombia. Acta Psychiatr Scand 76:561–567, 1987

McFarlane AC: Long-term psychiatric morbidity after a natural disaster. Med J Aust 145:561–563, 1986

McFarlane AC: The longitudinal course of posttraumatic morbidity: the range of outcomes and their predictors. J Nerv Ment Dis 176:30–39, 1988a

McFarlane AC: The phenomenology of post-traumatic stress disorders following a natural disaster. J Nerv Ment Dis 176:22–29, 1988b

Norris, FH: Towards establishing a data base for the prospective study of traumatic stress. Paper presented at National Institute of Mental Health workshop, June 1988. Traumatic stress: defining terms and instruments. Bethesda, MD, Uniformed Services University of the Health Sciences, June 1988

Norris F, Kaniasty K: Reliability of delayed self-reports in disaster research. J Trauma Stress 5:575–588, 1992

Parker G: Cyclone Tracy and Darwin evacuees: on the restoration of the species. Br J Psychiatry 130:548–555, 1977

Perry S, Difede J, Musngi G, et al: Predictors of posttraumatic stress disorder after burn injury. Am J Psychiatry 149:931–935, 1992

Quarentelli EL: An assessment of conflicting views on mental health: the consequences of traumatic events, in Trauma and its Wake. Edited by Figley CR. New York, Brunner/Mazel, 1985, pp 173–215

Robins LN, Helzer JE, Croughan J, et al: National Institute of Mental Health Diagnostic Interview Schedule: its history, characteristics, and validity. Arch Gen Psychiatry 38:381–389, 1981

Rosenheck R, Becnel H, Blank AS, et al: Returning Persian Gulf Troops: First Year Findings. Report of the Department of Veterans Affairs to the United States Congress on the Psychological Effects of the Persian Gulf War, 1992

Rubin CB, Nahavandian M: Details on Frequency of Disasters, Incidents for Federally Declared Disasters, 1965–1985. Washington, DC, George Washington University, Program in Science, Technology and Public Policy, 1987

Rundell JR, Ursano RJ, Holloway HC, et al: Psychiatric responses to trauma. Hosp Community Psychiatry 40:68–74, 1989

Shore JH, Tatum EL, Vollmer WM: Psychiatric reactions to disaster: the Mount St. Helens experience. Am J Psychiatry 143:590–595, 1986

Shore JH, Vollmer WM, Tatum EL: Community patterns of posttraumatic stress disorders. J Nerv Ment Dis 177:681–685, 1989

Sledge WH, Boydstun JA, Rahe AJ: Self-concept changes related to war captivity. Arch Gen Psychiatry 37:430–443, 1980

Smith E, North C: Posttraumatic stress disorder in natural disasters and technological accidents, in International Handbook of Traumatic Stress Syndromes. Edited by Wilson JP, Raphael B. New York, Plenum, 1993, pp 405–420

Smith EM, Robins, LN, Pryzbeck TR, et al: Psychosocial consequences of a disaster, in Disaster Stress Studies: New Methods and Findings. Edited by Shore J. Washington, DC, American Psychiatric Press, 1986, pp 50–76

Smith EM, North CS, McCool RE, et al: Acute post-disaster psychiatric disorders: identification of those at risk. Am J Psychiatry 147:202–206, 1989

Solomon SD, Smith EM, Robins LN, et al: Social involvement as a mediator of disaster-induced stress. Journal of Applied Social Psychology 17:1092–1112, 1987

Solomon SD, Gerrity ET, Muff AM: Efficacy of treatment for Posttraumatic Stress Disorder. JAMA 268:633–638, 1992

Solomon Z, Benbenishty R: The role of proximity, immediacy, and expectancy in frontline treatment of combat stress reaction among Israelis in the Lebanon War. Am J Psychiatry 143:613–617, 1986

Solomon Z, Mikulincer M: Combat stress reactions, posttraumatic stress disorder, and social adjustment: a study of Israeli veterans. J Nerv Ment Dis 175:277–285, 1987

Solomon Z, Mikulincer M, Kotler M: A two-year follow-up of somatic complaints among Israeli combat stress reaction casualties. J Psychosom Res 31:463–469, 1987

Spiegel D, Cardeña E: Disintegrated experience: the dissociative disorders revisited. J Abnorm Psychol 100:366–378, 1993

Steinglass P, Gerrity E: Natural disasters and post-traumatic stress disorder: short-term versus long-term recovery in two disaster-affected communities. Journal of Applied Social Psychology 20:1746–1765, 1990

Sutker PB, Winstead DK, Galina ZH, et al: Cognitive deficits and psychopathology among former prisoners of war and combat veterans of the Korean conflict. Am J Psychiatry 148:67–72, 1991

Taylor V: Good news about disaster. Psychology Today 11:93–94, 124–126, 1977

Titchener JL, Kapp FT: Family and character change at Buffalo Creek. Am J Psychiatry 133:295–299, 1976

Ursano RJ: The Vietnam-era prisoner of war: precaptivity personality and development of psychiatric illness. Am J Psychiatry 138:315–318, 1981

Ursano RJ: Comments on "Post-traumatic stress disorder: the stressor criterion." J Nerv Ment Dis 75:273–275, 1987

Ursano RJ, Fullerton CS: Cognitive and behavioral responses to trauma. Journal of Applied Social Psychology 20:1766–1775, 1990

Ursano RJ, McCarroll JE: The nature of the traumatic stressor: handling dead bodies. J Nerv Ment Dis 178:396–398, 1990

Ursano RJ, Boydstun JA, Wheatley RD: Psychiatric illness in U.S. Air Force Vietnam prisoners of war: a five-year follow-up. Am J Psychiatry 138:310–314, 1981

Ursano RJ, Fullerton CS, Kao T, et al: PTSD in community samples. Proceedings of the International Society for Traumatic Stress Studies, World Conference, Amsterdam, The Netherlands, June 1992a

Ursano RJ, Tzu-Cheg K, Fullerton CS: Posttraumatic stress disorder and meaning: structuring human chaos. J Nerv Ment Dis 180:756–759, 1992b

Ursano RJ, Fullerton CS, McCaughey BG: Trauma and disaster, in Individual and Community Responses to Trauma and Disaster: The Structure of Human Chaos. Edited by Ursano RJ, McCaughey BG, Fullerton CS. London, Cambridge University Press, 1994a, pp 3–27

Ursano RJ, McCaughey BG, Fullerton CS: Individual and Community Responses to Trauma and Disaster: The Structure of Human Chaos. London: Cambridge University Press, 1994b

Ursano RJ, Fullerton CS, Bhartiya V, et al: Longitudinal assessment of posttraumatic stress disorder and depression after exposure to traumatic death. J Nerv Ment Dis 183:36–43, 1995

van der Kolk BA, van der Hart O: Pierre Janet and the breakdown of adaptation in psychological trauma. Am J Psychiatry 146:1530–1540, 1989

Weisæth L: A study of behavioral responses to an industrial disaster. Acta Psychiatr Scand 80 (suppl):13–24, 1989a

Weisæth L: The stressors and the post-traumatic stress syndrome after an industrial disaster. Acta Psychiatr Scand 80 (suppl):25–37, 1989b

Weisæth L: Psychological and psychiatric aspects of technological disasters, in Individual and Community Responses to Trauma and Disaster: The Structure of Human Chaos. Edited by Ursano RJ, McCaughey BG, Fullerton CS. London, Cambridge University Press, 1994, pp 72–102

Weisæth L, Eitinger L: Posttraumatic stress phenomena: common themes across wars, disasters, and traumatic events, in International Handbook of Traumatic Stress Syndromes. Edited by Wilson JP, Raphael B. New York, Plenum, 1993, pp 69–77

Wilson JP, Raphael B (eds): International Handbook of Traumatic Stress Syndromes. New York, Plenum, 1993

Part II

Acute Responses to Trauma and Disaster

Chapter 2

Multiple Stressors Following a Disaster and Dissociative Symptoms

Cheryl Koopman, Ph.D., Catherine Classen, Ph.D., and David Spiegel, M.D.

D o stressful events lead to more stressful events? In this chapter, we explore factors in the immediate aftermath of a large disaster—the 1991 Oakland/Berkeley firestorm—that led to further life stressors. We examine two factors—the loss of a home in the firestorm and dissociative symptoms in the storm's immediate aftermath—to determine what relationships these two factors had to stressful life events occurring in the months following the firestorm.

By definition, a disaster imposes tremendous hardship. Deleterious effects extending beyond the immediate, visible effects—such as the destruction of houses—are less obvious, however. The burdens imposed by a disaster may be worsened because the disaster may start a sequence of events that set a person's life on a downward spiral.

Survivors must contend with a variety of hardships after a natural disaster. Some symbolic losses bring great psychological distress. For example, in the week immediately after the Oakland/Berkeley firestorm, one woman's grief focused on photographs of her great-grandparents, which were lost in the firestorm. She said, "You have no idea what this is like to actually go through." Hers was a personal

This research was supported by a contract with the Violence and Traumatic Stress Research Branch of the National Institute of Mental Health and by a grant from the John D. and Catherine T. MacArthur Foundation. We are grateful to Helena C. Kraemer for her help on the data analysis. We also wish to thank Bernard Baars, Dennis Barton, Susan Diamond, Robert Matano, Bita Nouriani, Susan Reaburn, Kristen Soika, and the Oakland/Berkeley firestorm survivors who participated in this research.

kind of loss resulting from the fire. Another kind of hardship many survivors contended with was the loss of their home (Solomon and Canino 1990).

The psychological impact of such losses can be interpreted within a model of stress known as *conservation of resources* (Hobfoll 1989). This model asserts that personal resources (e.g., shelter) and social resources (e.g., family roles such as homemaker) are integral to psychological well-being because they are tools that can be used to achieve desired states. Therefore, losing these kinds of resources is highly stressful. According to the conservation of resources model, the magnitude of loss of resources is the primary factor influencing psychological adjustment in the aftermath of a disaster.

Evidence supporting this model has come from research (Freedy et al. 1992) that found that resource loss in Hurricane Hugo was strongly related to psychological distress assessed in the third month after the disaster. One reason resource loss might lead to greater psychological distress is that losing resources leads to further stressful events that then create more psychological duress. We tested this idea by examining whether loss of a particular kind of resource—one's home—would be significantly likely to precipitate other kinds of stressful events.

Another consequence immediately following a disaster is the psychological distress experienced in response to the disaster. Researchers have identified a pattern of acute stress reactions (Madakasira and O'Brien 1987; Spiegel and Cardeña 1991) that includes symptoms of dissociation (Cardeña and Spiegel 1993; Hillman 1981; Lindemann 1944; McFarlane 1986; Noyes et al. 1977), anxiety (Dollinger 1985; McFarlane 1986; Titchener and Kapp 1976), avoidant behavior (North et al. 1989; Wilkinson 1983), and reexperiencing reminders of the trauma (Feinstein 1989; Wilkinson 1983). An extreme version of this pattern, known as acute stress disorder (ASD), appears in DSM-IV (American Psychiatric Association 1994).

The clinical significance and importance of ASD is underscored by systematic evidence that such symptoms are significantly related to later systems of posttraumatic stress disorder (Marmar et al. 1992; Rothblum et al. 1992). The dynamics of this relationship demand further investigation, however.

In this chapter, we focus on the relationship of dissociative symptoms experienced in the immediate aftermath of a disaster to later stressful events. We were particularly interested in the relationship of later events to dissociative symptoms. We wanted to extend the time frame of actions following the firestorm to examine whether dissociative symptoms in the firestorm's aftermath would show significant relationships to events in the long run.

METHODS

Overview

The Oakland/Berkeley firestorm began on October 20, 1991, and continued for 2 days, causing the deaths of 24 people and consuming 3,135 residences (Taylor and Wildermuth 1991). After obtaining approval for this study from our institutional human subjects review board, we distributed a survey to respondents in the Oakland/Berkeley area between October 24 and October 31, 1991. A total of 187 respondents completed the survey; 94% of these respondents returned the survey within 3 weeks. A follow-up mail survey was conducted 7 months after the firestorm, with 154 completed questionnaires returned, for a follow-up rate of 82%. Of these 154 completed questionnaires, 69% were completed by 8 months after the firestorm, 97% by 9 months, 99% by 10 months, and 100% by 11 months.

Sample

Participants were recruited from three sources, which we expected to vary in exposure to the firestorm. The follow-up assessments reflected this original sampling distribution.

- 94 participants (including 74 who responded to the follow-up mailing) were recruited in front of a one-stop government service center providing assistance to firestorm survivors and through personal contacts with people living in neighborhoods next to firestorm affected areas.
- 44 participants (including 36 follow-up respondents) were University of California–Berkeley students recruited from four fraternities

and sororities that had been evacuated during the firestorm.
- 49 participants (44 follow-up respondents) were graduate students recruited from the Wright Institute, a professional school of psychology in Berkeley, which was not evacuated.

Measures

Demographic characteristics. Demographic characteristics were assessed by self-report survey questions on gender, age, education, and city of residence.

Losing home or apartment. Respondents were asked whether the firestorm had destroyed their home and recorded their response as "Yes" or "No."

Dissociative symptoms in the firestorm's immediate aftermath. A study of acute stress reactions to the 1989 Loma Prieta earthquake (Cardeña and Spiegel 1993) used an earlier version of the Stanford Acute Stress Reaction Questionnaire (SASRQ); we used a revised version (Classen et al. 1991) to assess dissociative symptoms in the aftermath of the Oakland/Berkeley firestorm. The version we used contained 33 self-report items representing five domains of dissociative symptoms: amnesia (six items), depersonalization (nine items), derealization (nine items), psychic numbing (four items), and stupor (five items). Subjects recorded their responses on a six-point Likert scale to indicate the frequency with which they experienced each symptom during and since the firestorm—from 0 = "not experienced" to 5 = "very often experienced." C. Classen and D. Spiegel (Unpublished manuscript, September 1992) found that this measure has high internal consistency (total dissociative symptoms, Cronbach's alpha = .90), as well as concurrent validity (r = .62-.63, P < .001) with the intrusion and avoidance subscales of the Impact of Event Scale (Horowitz et al. 1979).

Because we were interested in determining the number of dissociative symptoms each subject experienced, we dichotomized the responses on the dissociative symptoms scale of the SASRQ so that responses of 3 = "sometimes experienced" or above were recoded as a 1 and responses of 2 = "rarely experienced" or less were recoded as a 0. For each of the five symptoms, we counted occurrence if at least one item tapping the symptom received a score of 1; we then summed the occurrence of each of the five symptoms for a total dissociative symptom score of 0–5.

Schedule of Recent Experience. The Schedule of Recent Experience (Holmes and Rahe 1967) assesses the incidence of 42 stressful events in a given time period—which in our study was the interlude from the firestorm to the follow-up assessment (7 to 11 months). Respondents were asked to record the number of times, if any, each event had occurred during this period. Sample items included: "minor violations of the law (e.g., traffic tickets, jaywalking, disturbing the peace, etc.)" and "divorce." Responses may be multiplied by a point value indicating the overall stress level. We did not make this further transformation of the data; however, instead we dichotomized the responses because in this study we were interested simply in whether the event had occurred since the firestorm.

Civilian version of the Mississippi Scale for posttraumatic stress disorder. We drew two other events from the civilian version of the Mississippi Scale (Keane et al. 1987, 1988), which we included in the 7-month follow-up assessment to measure posttraumatic stress symptoms in reference to combat-related stress. We adapted this instrument for our purposes by rewording the Likert-style statements to refer to "the firestorm" as the traumatic event. Responses on the Mississippi Scale are indicated as levels of agreement/disagreement on a scale of 1–5. The two items of interest in this study were, "There have been times when I used alcohol (or other drugs) to help me sleep or to make me forget about things that happened in the firestorm" and "Before the firestorm, I had more close friends than I have now." We scored responses of 3 = "sometimes" or greater as indicating occurrence.

Data Analysis

We computed descriptive statistics on the loss of a home in the firestorm, dissociative symptoms, and total number of stressful life events assessed on the Schedule of Recent Experience. We computed frequencies for each event assessed on the Schedule of Recent Experience to determine the type of analysis to conduct on it. We conducted logistic regression analysis on events that had occurred in less than

25% of the sample and multiple regression analysis on events that had occurred in 25% or more of the sample; we used the stepwise forward procedure in both kinds of analysis to examine whether dissociative symptoms or the loss of a home—the two independent variables—showed a stronger relationship to later stressful life events.

RESULTS

Of the 154 respondents who completed both the initial survey and the 7-month follow-up assessment, 62% were female; the respondents' mean age was 36.1 years (SD = 12.8), and their mean number of years of education was 16.8 (SD = 2.9). All of the subjects had been exposed to the firestorm; 83% of the respondents lived in Oakland or Berkeley at the time of the firestorm.

Thirty-four of the 154 participants (22%) had lost their homes in the firestorm. Respondents reported on the Schedule of Recent Experience a mean of 2.4 dissociative symptoms (SD = 1.8) during and immediately following the firestorm and a mean of 5.3 stressful life events (SD = 4.6). Table 2–1 presents the percentage of respondents who reported the occurrence of each event during the 7- to 11-month follow-up interval.

On the civilian version of the Mississippi Scale, 12% of the respondents reported using alcohol or drugs to sleep or forget, and 13% reported having fewer close friends. The total number of stressful life events was significantly related to the number of dissociative symptoms (R^2 = .11, F [df = 1, 152] = 20.31, P < .0001) and, secondarily, to the loss of one's home in the firestorm (R^2 = .04, F [df = 2, 151] = 7.59, P < .0001). These relationships are illustrated in Figure 2–1; dissociative symptoms are dichotomized at the median for ease of presentation.

We found some statistically significant relationships between specific kinds of events and the loss of a home and dissociative symptoms. Table 2–2 presents percentages of respondents experiencing each kind of event that was significantly related to loss of home or to dissociative symptoms, analyzed by those who did or did not lose their home and by those who experienced fewer than or more than the median number of dissociative symptoms.

Table 2–1. Percentage of respondents reporting each event's occurrence after the firestorm

Event	Percentage reporting
1. A lot more or a lot less trouble with the boss	15
2. A major change in sleeping habits (sleeping a lot more or a lot less, or change in part of day when asleep)	39
3. A major change in eating habits (a lot more or a lot less food intake, or very different meal hours or surroundings)	29
4. A revision of personal habits (dress, manners, associations, etc.)	21
5. A major change in your usual type and/or amount of recreation	34
6. A major change in your social activities (e.g., clubs, dancing, movies, visiting, etc.)	24
7. A major change in church activities (e.g., a lot more or a lot less than usual)	7
8. A major change in number of family get-togethers (e.g., a lot more or a lot less than usual)	18
9. A major change in financial state (e.g., a lot worse off or a lot better off than usual)	35
10. Trouble with in-laws	5
11. A major change in the number of arguments with spouse (e.g., either a lot more or a lot less than usual regarding child rearing, personal habits, etc.)	15
12. Sexual difficulties	13
13. Major personal injury or illness	10
14. Death of a close family member (other than spouse)	5
15. Death of a spouse	1
16. Death of a close friend	10
17. Gaining a new family member (e.g., through birth, adoption, oldster moving in, etc.)	10
18. Major change in the health or behavior of a family member	20
19. Change in residence	39

(continued)

Table 2–1. Percentage of respondents reporting each event's occurrence after the firestorm *(continued)*

Event	Percentage reporting
20. Detention in jail or other institution	0
21. Minor violations of the law (e.g., traffic tickets, jaywalking, disturbing the peace, etc)	17
22. Major business readjustment (e.g., merger, reorganization, bankruptcy, etc.)	14
23. Marriage	0
24. Divorce	2
25. Marital separation from spouse	3
26. Outstanding personal achievement	36
27. Son or daughter leaving home (e.g., marriage, attending college, etc.)	4
28. Retirement from work	3
29. Major change in working hours or conditions	42
30. Major change in responsibilities at work (e.g., promotion, demotion, lateral transfer)	27
31. Being fired from work	2
32. Major change in living conditions (e.g., building a new home, remodeling, deterioration of home or neighborhood)	26
33. Wife/husband beginning or ceasing work outside the home	7
34. Taking out a mortgage or loan for a major purchase (e.g., purchasing a home, business, etc.)	14
35. Taking out a mortgage or loan for a lesser purchase (e.g., purchasing a car, TV, freezer, etc.)	12
36. Foreclosure on a mortgage or a loan	1
37. Vacation	51
38. Changing to a new school	3
39. Changing to a different line of work	13
40. Beginning or ceasing formal schooling	16
41. Marital reconciliation with mate	1
42. Pregnancy	2

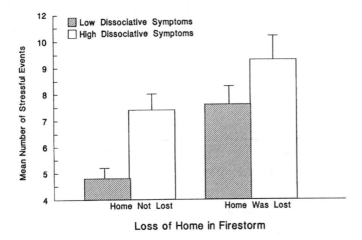

Figure 2–1. Mean number of stressful life events, analyzed by loss of home and dissociative symptoms.

Loss of Home

Subsequent events that we found were significantly related to losing a home in the firestorm included major change in financial state (F [df = 1, 152] = 28.31, $P < .0001$); change in residence (F [df = 1, 152] = 73.14, $P < .0001$); major change in living conditions (F [df = 1, 152] = 18.24, $P < .0001$); major business readjustment (Wald [df = 1] = 13.50, $P < .0002$); taking out a mortgage or loan (Wald [df = 1] = 4.97, $P < .05$); outstanding personal achievement (F [df = 1, 152] = 6.81, $P < .01$); major change in family get-togethers (Wald [df = 1] = 5.58, $P < .02$); revision of personal habits (dress, manners, associations, etc.) (Wald [df = 1] = 10.16, $P < .002$); and minor violations of the law (Wald [df = 1] = 8.76, $P < .01$]. There also was a statistically significant relationship between the loss of a home and using alcohol or drugs (Wald [df = 1] = 3.35, $P < .07$).

Dissociative Symptoms

Subsequent events that we found were significantly related to dissociative symptoms included major personal illness or injury (Wald [df = 1] = 6.21, $P < .02$); major change in eating habits (F [df = 1, 152] = 15.01, $P < .0002$); major change in sleeping habits (F [df = 1, 152] = 38.32,

Table 2–2. Percentage of respondents reporting events occurrence after the firestorm, analyzed by loss of home or dissociative symptoms, if statistically significant

Event	Percentage reporting	
	Did not lose home ($n = 120$)	Did lose home ($n = 34$)
Change in residence	24	91
Major change in living conditions	18	53
Taking out a mortgage or a loan	11	27
Major change in financial state	25	71
Major business readjustment	8	35
Outstanding personal achievement	42	18
Major change in family get-togethers	14	32
Revision in personal habits	15	41
Minor violations of the law	13	35
Using alcohol/drugs to sleep or to forget the firestorm	7	17
	Low dissociation ($n = 82$)	High dissociation ($n = 72$)
Major personal injury or illness	5	15
Major change in eating habits	18	40
Major change in sleeping habits	20	61
Major change in type/amount of recreation	28	40
Major change in social activities	13	36
Major change in church activities	2	13
Having fewer close friends	5	22

$P < .0001$); major change in type/amount of recreation (F [df = 1, 152] = 4.97, $P < .05$); major change in social activities (Wald [df = 11] = 8.24, $P < .005$]; major change in church activities (Wald [df = 1] = 7.02, $P < .01$); and having fewer close friends (Wald [df = 1] = 13.97, $P < .0002$). No other events were significantly related to dissociative symptoms.

DISCUSSION

Our results show that people who experience a major disaster, such as the Oakland/Berkeley firestorm, continue to experience many stressful changes in the months that follow. Although some of these changes relate directly to physical damage from the disaster (i.e., losing one's home), other changes relate more to the intrapsychic consequences of coping with the disaster (i.e., dissociative symptoms) than to physical damage. These findings have several implications.

First, people who survive a natural disaster are at risk of continuing to experience life events that further exacerbate their stress. Thus, not only do disaster survivors need psychological help to cope with stress in the immediate aftermath of a disaster, but also many of these persons are likely to undergo further stressors in the next few months for which they may need additional help and support. This finding has implications for the identification of persons who are at risk for becoming overwhelmed with stress; simply examining a disaster's immediate consequences will not provide an obvious indication of how much stress an individual will experience in subsequent months.

Second, people who lose a home in a disaster are likely to continue to experience a series of stressful life changes. Persons who lose their home must move into new residences, often make major changes in their residences (e.g., remodeling), and are likely to take out a mortgage or loan—perhaps to pay for their move and home remodeling, as well as major new furnishings to replace those lost when the home was destroyed. Although such changes follow predictably from the loss of a home, they may have greater significance: They form a larger, cascading pattern of stressful events that may overwhelm disaster survivors beyond the initial stress of losing their home.

The conservation of resources model (Hobfoll 1989) predicts that these changes, which are stressful in the short run (Holmes and Rahe 1967), will replenish the diminished resources of those who lose their homes and therefore lead to less stress in the long run. Research on coping behavior after a disaster (reviewed in Gibbs 1989), which affirms that active problem-solving coping behavior improves the psychological well-being of disaster survivors, also predicts long-term benefits from these actions.

In contrast, other events that we found were significantly related to the loss of a home are unlikely to decrease stress in the long run. These events include the lower likelihood of experiencing an outstanding personal achievement, the greater likelihood of committing minor violations of the law, and the trend toward greater use of alcohol or drugs to aid in sleep or to forget the disaster.

People who lose a home also are more likely to experience a major change in family get-togethers. One of the participants in this study who lost her home described her family's altered lifestyle:

> Within a week after the fire, we were offered the use of a furnished house owned by a member of our church. To stock the kitchen we bought grocery staples, including a dozen eggs. Over a month later we still hadn't used a single one of those eggs. There was never time to sit together for a cooked breakfast. Every day there were urgent matters to attend to. Days off from work were taken up with insurance and neighborhood association meetings. Sundays became household shopping days.

A revision in personal habits also relates to the loss of a home. The woman quoted above also described how she used to worry about her body weight, having lost her bathroom scale and all her old clothes; however, she no longer gives it a second thought.

Perhaps the most striking results of this study concern our findings of significant relationships between dissociative symptoms experienced in the immediate aftermath of the disaster and stressful life changes occurring in the months after the firestorm. One finding may have important health implications: People who experience more dissociative symptoms are significantly more likely than those experiencing fewer dissociative symptoms to experience a major injury or illness in the months that follow; they also are more likely than others to experience major changes in eating and sleeping habits—both of which may affect their health. Furthermore, their relationships with other persons are more likely to be disrupted, as self-reports of fewer friends since the firestorm and major changes in social, recreational, and church activities showed. Psychiatrists increasingly understand minor violations of the law and possibly increased drinking or drug use as posttraumatic stress responses.

Explanations for relationships between dissociative symptoms and later major illness or injury, having fewer friends, and major changes in eating and sleeping habits are less apparent. For example, dissociative symptoms assessed in a disaster's immediate aftermath may persist among many survivors, indicating that these individuals do not pay adequate attention to their health routines and their environments, which leads to greater illness and injury and disruptions in eating and sleeping. Alternatively, dissociative symptoms may be part of a pattern of psychobiological trauma responses (van der Kolk and Greenberg 1987), in which survivors become addicted to high-risk events involving traumatic reexposure (such as driving fast, as they may have had to at the time of the fire), which increases their likelihood of injury or illness.

Perhaps dissociative symptoms distract some survivors from attending to their interpersonal relationships, resulting in the loss of some friendships. The quality, more than the quantity, of interpersonal relations may deteriorate among persons high in dissociative symptoms, so that they are unable to experience their usual intensity of connection with other persons. Just as dissociation may serve as an adaptive defense against trauma as it is occurring (Cardeña and Spiegel 1993; Spiegel and Cardeña 1991), it also may desensitize people to danger.

We do not have enough information to evaluate alternative explanations for the relationships we found between loss of home and dissociative symptoms in the immediate aftermath of a fire with continued stressful events over the following months. Understanding the causal links would help psychiatrists to design interventions targeting trauma survivors. Future research should examine how the short-term consequences of a disaster, such as losing a home and experiencing dissociative symptoms, lead to further stressful changes in the long term. Investigators also need to identify critical decision points where intervention can be most effective in ensuring that disaster survivors steer their lives as much as possible toward changes that support physical health, alleviate emotional distress, and enhance interpersonal relationships.

REFERENCES

American Psychiatric Association: Diagnostic and Statistical Manual of Mental Disorders, 4th Edition. Washington, DC, American Psychiatric Association, 1994

Cardeña E, Spiegel D: Dissociative reactions to the Bay Area earthquake. Am J Psychiatry 150:474–478, 1993

Classen C, Cardeña E, Spiegel D: Acute Stress Reaction Questionnaire. Department of Psychiatry and Behavioral Sciences, Stanford Medical School, 1991

Dollinger SJ: Lightning-strike disaster among children. Br J Med Psychol 58:375–383, 1985

Feinstein A: Posttraumatic stress disorder: a descriptive study supporting DSM-III-R criteria. Am J Psychiatry 146:665–666, 1989

Freedy JR, Shaw DL, Jarrell MP, et al: Towards an understanding of the psychological impact of natural disasters: an application of the conservation resources stress model. J Trauma Stress 5:441–454, 1992

Gibbs MS: Factors in the victim that mediate between disaster and psychopathology: a review. J Trauma Stress 2:489–514, 1989

Hillman RB: The psychopathology of being held hostage. Am J Psychiatry 138:1193–1197, 1981

Hobfoll SE: Conservation of resources: a new attempt at conceptualizing stress. Am Psychol 44:513–524, 1989

Holmes TH, Rahe RH: The Social Readjustment Rating Scale. J Psychosom Res 11:213–218, 1967

Horowitz MJ, Wilner N, Alvarez W: Impact of Event Scale: a measure of subjective distress. Psychosom Med 41:209–218, 1979

Keane TM, Caddell JM, Taylor KL: Posttraumatic stress disorder: evidence for diagnostic validity and methods of psychological assessment. J Clin Psychol 43:32–43, 1987

Keane TM, Caddell JM, Taylor KL: Mississippi Scale for combat-related posttraumatic stress disorder: three studies in reliability and validity. J Consult Clin Psychol 56:85–90, 1988

Lindemann E: Symptomatology and management of acute grief. Am J Psychiatry 101:141–148, 1944

Madakasira S, O'Brien KF: Acute posttraumatic stress disorder in victims of a natural disaster. J Nerv Ment Dis 175:286–290, 1987

Marmar C, Weiss D, Schlanger W, et al: Peritraumatic dissociation and posttraumatic stress disorder. Paper presented at the International Society of Traumatic Stress Studies, October 1992

McFarlane AC: Posttraumatic morbidity of a disaster. J Nerv Ment Dis 174: 4–14, 1986

North CS, Smith EM, McCool RE, et al: Acute postdisaster coping and adjustment. J Trauma Stress 2:353–360, 1989

Noyes R, Hoenk PR, Kuperman S, et al: Depersonalization in accident victims and psychiatric patients. J Nerv Ment Dis 164:401–407, 1977

Rothblum BO, Foa EB, Riggs DS, et al: A prospective examination of post-traumatic stress disorder in rape victims. J Trauma Stress 5:455–475, 1992

Solomon SD, Canino GJ: Appropriateness of DSM-III-R criteria for post-traumatic stress disorder. Compr Psychiatry 31:227–237, 1990

Spiegel D, Cardeña E: Disintegrated experience: the dissociative disorders revisited. J Abnorm Psychol 100:366–378, 1991

Taylor M, Wildermuth J: It was worst wildfire in US history. San Francisco Chronicle, October 25, 1991, p A1

Titchener JL, Kapp FT: Family and character change at Buffalo Creek. Am J Psychiatry 133:295–299, 1976

van der Kolk BA, Greenberg MS: The psychobiology of the trauma response: hyperarousal, constriction, and addiction to traumatic reexposure in psychological trauma, in Psychological Trauma. Edited by van der Kolk BA. Washington, DC, American Psychiatric Press, 1987, pp 63–87

Wilkinson CB: Aftermath of a disaster: the collapse of the Hyatt Regency Hotel skywalks. Am J Psychiatry 140:1134–1139, 1983

Chapter 3

Exposure to Traumatic Death in Disaster and War

James E. McCarroll, Ph.D., Robert J. Ursano, M.D., and Carol S. Fullerton, Ph.D.

The sight of a large number of bodies is frequently described as over-whelming—even for the most experienced rescue worker. "The bodies just kept coming and coming. It felt like I was surrounded. It's hard not to look at the bodies when they are surrounding you. I looked around and saw 15 dead bodies looking at me with their jaws cut open" (Ursano and McCarroll 1994, p. 54).

The likelihood of violent death and the presence of human remains—burned, dismembered, mutilated, or relatively intact—is common to nearly all disasters, combat, and other cataclysmic events. Body recovery, identification, transport, and burial involve pro-longed contact with mass death. Repeated exposure to traumatic death puts disaster workers at risk for the development of posttrau-matic stress (Green et al. 1983; Jones 1985; McCarroll et al. 1993d; Paton 1994; Raphael 1986; Short 1979; Taylor and Frazer 1982).

Exposure to traumatic death is a potent psychological stressor (Bolin 1985; Green 1993; Lifton 1967; Sutker et al. 1994a, 1994b; Ursano and McCarroll 1994). Posttraumatic stress responses are common at a sufficient level of impairment; however, traumatic stress symp-toms may suggest a psychiatric disorder. Although systematic re-search on the psychiatric effects of trauma and disaster increased dramatically with the introduction of posttraumatic stress disorder (PTSD) in DSM-III (American Psychiatric Association 1980), indi-vidual and group preparation for, behavior during, and response after witnessing traumatic death have received little scientific scru-tiny (for comprehensive collections of research on trauma, disas-ters, and combat, see Ursano et al. 1994; Wilson and Raphael 1993).

In this chapter, we review the changing structure of PTSD and the epidemiology of trauma and PTSD. We examine the relationship between traumatic stress and grotesque death, including anticipatory stress and exposure to traumatic death in Vietnam, the 1989 invasion of Panama (Operation Just Cause), and the Persian Gulf War (Operation Desert Storm).

THE CHANGING STRUCTURE OF POSTTRAUMATIC STRESS DISORDERS

Scope of the Diagnosis

Early observations of posttraumatic stress began with descriptions of soldier breakdown in war. During the Civil War, for example, observers used the term "nostalgia" to describe the symptoms of combat stress. Terms such as "shell shock," "battle fatigue," and "war neurosis" were common descriptors of emotional responses during World War I (Trimble 1981). The "thousand-mile stare" described the wearied soldier on the verge of collapse. Stress symptoms following combat exposure include anxiety, startle reactions, and numbness (Grinker and Spiegel 1945). Clinicians and researchers also have described traumatic stress responses following other catastrophic events including concentration camp survivors (Chodoff 1963; Etinger and Strom 1973; Krystal 1968) and rescue workers following the Hiroshima devastation (Lifton 1967).

PTSD was introduced as a psychiatric diagnosis in DSM-III. Since its inception, PTSD has been and continues to be the subject of much debate (e.g., Andreasen 1985; Davidson and Foa 1993; Gunderson and Sabo 1993; Smith and North 1993; Weisæth and Eitinger 1993; Wolfe and Keane 1993). Nevertheless, the inclusion of PTSD in DSM-III represented an important link between the framers of psychiatric nomenclature and the clinicians who cared for Vietnam veterans and requested recognition of a post-Vietnam syndrome (Helzer et al. 1987; Laufer et al. 1985a, 1985b).

DSM-III-R (American Psychiatric Association 1987) refined the diagnostic criteria for PTSD by defining the stressor criterion operationally and describing symptoms in a broader range of populations (e.g., traumatized children). DSM-IV (American Psychiatric Association 1994) broadened the scope of responses to traumatic events with the new diagnosis *acute stress disorder* (ASD); ASD symptoms occur within 4 weeks of a traumatic event and last between 2 days and 4 weeks. Systematic empirical investigation of ASD is just beginning (Davidson and Foa 1993; Spiegel and Cardeña 1991).

Although PTSD has been the most studied traumatic disorder in recent years, it is not the only psychiatric disorder that follows traumatic events. Many psychiatric disorders are associated with trauma, including major depression, generalized anxiety disorder, substance abuse, somatization, and adjustment disorder (Davidson and Fairbank 1993; Green et al. 1992; Karam 1991; Keane and Wolfe 1990; Kulka et al. 1990; McFarlane 1993; Rundell et al. 1989; Smith and North 1993).

The stressor criterion: challenge and controversy.   The severity, nature, and duration of the stressor are primary risk factors for the development of PTSD. Several aspects of the stressor have been associated with posttraumatic stress—for example, threat to life, physical injury, loss of home, death, and exposure to the grotesque (Green 1990, 1993; March 1993). This analysis only begins the definition; however, the interaction of the nature of the stressor and its mediators determines the individual's experience of traumatic stress.

The stressor criterion controversy centers on whether psychiatrists consider an experience a stressor because an individual perceives it to be traumatic (Breslau and Davis 1987; Solomon and Canino 1990) or define the stressor objectively (Norris 1992). Breslau and Davis (1987) cautioned that the DSM-III stressor criterion should be limited to an *extraordinary* event and suggested the consideration of *ordinary* stressors as meeting the diagnostic criterion for PTSD. Moreover, personal characteristics of the individual (vulnerability) and the nature of the social environment (support) modify posttraumatic responses across types of stressors.

Responding to Breslau and Davis (1987), Horowitz et al. (1987), Lindy et al. (1987), and Ursano (1987) noted that there is ample evidence for the association of extraordinary stressors and PTSD. These authors reviewed studies showing that the quantity of stress was consistently associated with breakdown. Ursano (1987) also noted that although the diagnosis of PTSD requires a stressor quantity, it does not exclude issues relating to the quality of the stressor.

Epidemiology of Trauma and PTSD

Recent studies have examined the prevalence of PTSD in the general population and in persons exposed to natural and technological disasters, accidents, and combat (see Davidson and Foa 1993; Green 1994). Examinations of the epidemiology of trauma and PTSD have become more accurate since the standardization of diagnostic measures such as the Structured Clinical Interview (SCID) for DSM-III-R (Spitzer et al. 1987) and the Diagnostic Interview Schedule (DIS) (Helzer and Robins 1988), which was used in the Epidemiologic Catchment Area (ECA) (e.g., Baum et al. 1993; Green 1990; Kulka and Schlenger 1993; Weiss 1993). Taking into account a number of broad-based epidemiological studies of trauma and PTSD (e.g., Breslau and Davis 1992; Breslau et al. 1991; Davidson and Smith 1990; Helzer et al. 1987; Kilpatrick and Resnick 1993; Kulka et al. 1991; Norris 1992), Green (1994) estimated that approximately 75% of all Americans will be exposed to a traumatic event sometime during their lives; 25% of those exposed to a traumatic event (Criterion A, DSM-III-R) will develop PTSD.

Systematic examination of *acute* responses to trauma has been limited by the absence of standardized diagnostic criteria. Estimates of the prevalence of posttraumatic stress disorders and symptoms have not included what may be the largest group of people exposed to trauma: those with symptoms lasting only several days to a few weeks after the trauma. Investigations of acute responses to trauma have begun, however (Davidson and Foa 1993; Spiegel and Cardeña 1991), and DSM-IV's introduction of ASD as a diagnosis has provided added impetus.

PTSD and traumatic death: community studies.   Norris (1992) studied the impact of 10 traumatic events in a sample of 1,000 adults. A lifetime prevalence of 30.2% for tragic death was reported; the prevalence was equal in men and women but higher among whites than blacks. Seeing someone killed or seriously hurt was associated with PTSD in 23.6% of the cases and was among the traumatic events that produced higher rates among exposed women than men. The rate of crime-related PTSD among women (12%) was twice that of men (6%).

PTSD in veterans. Exposure to combat and abusive violence in veterans are strong predictors of PTSD (see Foy et al. 1984; Lee et al. 1995; March 1993). In a national study of male Vietnam combat veterans, Kulka et al. (1990) found PTSD rates to be 31% lifetime and 15% current; in female veterans, PTSD rates were 27% lifetime and 9% current. The incidence of psychiatric disorders after combat is positively associated with the degree of war trauma experienced, witnessing/participation in atrocities, and being wounded (Kulka et al. 1990, 1991; Sutker et al. 1994a; Ursano et al. 1981).

PTSD in victims of disaster and crime. Green et al. (1990a) studied survivors of the Buffalo Creek disaster and found that the rates of PTSD were 44% at 18–26 months after the disaster and 28% at 14 years after the disaster. Rates of PTSD in flood victims examined by Steinglass and Gerrity (1990) were 14.5% at 4 months and 4.5% at 16 months after the disaster. Steinglass and Gerrity (1990) also found PTSD in 21% of the population of one community 16 months after a tornado struck the area.

In a community study (*N* = 214), Kilpatrick et al. (1989, 1990) found that 29% of adult family members who were survivors of criminal homicide experienced PTSD after the loss. Using a modified DIS phone interview, Kilpatrick et al. (1987) found PTSD prevalence rates of 7.5% in women (*N* = 391) who had been criminally assaulted approximately 15 years earlier. A study of civilian trauma in a nationally representative sample of women (Resnick et al. 1993) reported a lifetime exposure to any type of traumatic event of 69%, with a lifetime prevalence of PTSD of 12.3% and a current rate of 4.6%.

PTSD AND GROTESQUE DEATH

Rescue workers are traumatized through the senses: viewing, smelling, and touching, experiencing the grotesque. Following a mass-casualty airplane crash, a disaster worker shut his eyes to go to sleep and saw one of the dead bodies from the crash. Many firefighters continued to smell the burning flesh long after they had gone home. Some washed repeatedly to get rid of the smell, but to no avail (Ursano and McCarroll 1994, pp. 65–66).

The association between exposure to traumatic death and post-traumatic stress responses has been examined in a wide range of trauma and disasters including combat (Appel 1966; Sutker et al. 1994b; Ursano and McCarroll 1990), airplane disasters (Bartone et al. 1989; Fullerton et al. 1992; McCarroll et al. 1993d; Taylor and Frazer 1982), earthquakes in Armenia (Paton 1994) and San Francisco (McCaughey et al. 1994), floods (Green et al. 1990a), tornadoes (Hershiser and Quarentelli 1976), fires (Green et al. 1983), volcano eruptions (Shore et al. 1986), mass suicides/cult deaths (Jones 1985; McCarroll et al. 1994), and disasters at sea (Alexander and Wells 1991; Holen 1993; Ursano et al. 1995). Taylor and Frazer (1982) reported that about a third of the volunteers who recovered bodies from the Mount Erebus air crash in Antarctica experienced transient problems of moderate to severe intensity. At 3 months, one-fifth of the volunteers continued to report high levels of stress-related symptoms. In a survey of 592 U.S. Air Force personnel involved in the recovery, transport, and identification of bodies of the Jonestown, Guyana, mass suicide, Jones (1985) found that youth, inexperience, lower rank, and greater exposure to the dead were associated with higher levels of emotional distress. Higher rates of dysphoria were found in blacks than whites, possibly because of greater identification with the black victims.

Ursano et al. (1995) examined acute and chronic posttraumatic stress in volunteer body handlers at 1, 4, and 13 months following a gun turret explosion aboard the USS *Iowa* that caused the deaths of 47 crew members. Probable PTSD was determined using the Impact of Event Scale (IES) (Horowitz et al. 1979), the Zung Depression Scale (Zung 1965), the revised Symptom Checklist (SCL-90-R) (Derogatis 1983), and additional PTSD criteria from DSM-III-R. Remains handlers had elevated intrusive and avoidant symptoms at 1, 4, and 13 months compared with those who did not work with the dead. Rates of PTSD symptoms among remains handlers declined over time, from 11% at 4 months after the disaster to 5% at 13 months after the disaster. In addition to increasing the risk of PTSD, exposure to traumatic death in this sample was associated with symptoms of intrusion, avoidance, hostility, and somatization that persisted for at least 1 year after the disaster.

Anticipation of Exposure to Grotesque Death

For some groups, anticipation of exposure to violent death may contribute to a stress response. The stress that actually occurs before the fact (before actual exposure) is *anticipatory stress*; the stress that a person thinks he or she may feel at the time stress actually occurs is *anticipated stress*. Studies of pilots in training for an unaccustomed mission found that anticipatory stress was greater in magnitude than the actual stress of the flight itself (Demos et al. 1969). In another study (Fenz and Epstein 1967), novice parachutists showed a sharp rise in physiological activity before a jump, whereas experienced persons produced an inverted U-shaped stress curve (low immediately before the jump); this reaction may represent an adaptive mechanism for the mastery of threat.

Anticipatory stress also produced heart rate acceleration in subjects performing public speaking (Penzien et al. 1982). Anticipation of surgery was associated with physiological stress (Corenblum and Taylor 1981) and hypoxic stress (Mefferd and Wieland 1966). Mefferd and Wieland (1966) found a negative relationship between levels of sympathetic nervous activity and performance on a psychometric test battery; thus, anticipation carried over into the actual stress period.

Anticipation of working with bodies following traumatic death is thought to be a powerful stressor (e.g., among firefighters; Ersland et al. 1989). McCarroll et al. (1993c) found gender and experience differences among military men and women who were asked to rate the stress they thought they would feel in handling the dead in 13 different situations. The situational variables related to locations in which remains would be recovered (e.g., battlefield conditions), the state of the remains (e.g., burned or decomposed), and personal characteristics of the bodies (someone known, a child, etc.). Anticipated stress was higher in inexperienced persons than in experienced persons, and women had higher levels of anticipated stress than men. Yet, men and women had similar responses to situations associated with the highest anticipated stress—handling the body of a friend, someone known, or a child. The lowest stress level applied to recovering the body of an enemy soldier. Variables related to the state of the remains (burned, mutilated, decomposed, or dismembered) led to anticipated stress levels between the two extremes.

A factor analysis of subject ratings produced three underlying constructs: the gruesomeness of the remains, the "emotional involvement" of the viewer with the remains, and possible threats to the remains handler (McCarroll et al. 1995). The gruesomeness factor accounted for the most variance (approximately 60% in men and women); emotional involvement accounted for 9% of the variance in men and 6% in women, and personal threat factors accounted for 7% of the variance in men and 14% in women. Gruesomeness was correlated with age (.11) and race (.21)—with nonwhites showing higher levels of stress than whites—and emotional attachment was negatively correlated with age (–.18).

The constructs identified by McCarroll et al. (1995) are important to the development of prevention programs; training and education could be directed toward the three stress factors. For example, a desensitization program that provides "inoculation" through the gradual introduction of morbid material and the teaching of cognitive strategies for focusing attention away from gruesome thoughts (see Meichenbaum 1977, for example) seems likely to be beneficial in reducing stress. Remains handlers have reported that looking at the faces and hands of the dead, seeing personal effects, and watching television reports that describe the dead and their families are highly stressful (McCarroll et al. 1993d); restricting their exposure to these situations may decrease their emotional attachment. Paying attention to one's own safety and following established medical procedures for working with remains that might carry diseases such as AIDS, hepatitis, and tuberculosis is most likely to reduce the third dimension of stress (personal threat).

McCarroll et al. (1993b) studied anticipatory stress in two groups working in the Operation Desert Storm mortuary before the arrival of the dead: those who would handle remains (mortuary workers) and those who would not (a group of support workers). These groups were mixtures of volunteers and nonvolunteers as well as persons with and without experience in handling the dead. The investigators used the Brief Symptom Inventory (Derogatis and Melisaratos 1983) to measure psychiatric distress. The mortuary workers had higher levels of pre-exposure distress than support workers; nonvolunteer mortuary workers had higher levels of distress than volunteers. Experienced mortuary workers reported fewer intrusive and avoidant symptoms than did inexperienced workers. Female mortuary workers had higher levels of distress than men, although the difference was slight. Inexperienced, nonvolunteer mortuary workers were at highest risk for generalized distress as well as intrusive and avoidant symptoms.

There may be circumstances in which anticipatory anxiety may be adaptive—that is, as a motivating or orienting part of adaptive function. Thus, anxiety reduction strategies may be helpful in some situations and harmful in others. The relationships among anticipatory stress, anticipated stress, and actual stress related to handling remains involve a complex system of variables.

Although studies of anticipated stress are valuable, the relationship between anticipated stress and actual stress has not been established. Most people appear to be aware of situations that disturb them and make efforts to avoid such situations; therefore, one would expect a high correlation between anticipated and actual stress. Studies on whether reducing anticipatory anxiety will reduce traumatization if another traumatic exposure occurs are needed. The effectiveness of specific coping strategies, such as those mentioned earlier, in reducing psychological symptoms also remains to be evaluated.

Grotesque Death in War

A Vietnam war veteran described:

> The most difficult for me was dealing with a body that had a single gunshot wound. We keyed in on the face of that person. We knew he was going home and his body would be viewable. This is more difficult than an air crash where the remains are severely charred or decomposed. If there isn't a face or a head, the whole focal point of expression is gone. In the case of a single shrapnel wound to the neck, we knew he was going home, out of the war, because of a single piece of metal—a fragment. It bothered me to see how sensitive life was to foreign objects compared to a hell of a crash or an explosion which leaves the dead unrecognizable. (Ursano and McCarroll 1994, p. 53)

In war, soldiers frequently witness the death or injury of other combatants (including comrades) and live under constant threat to their own life. War also entails instances in which civilians are killed and bodies are mutilated. Exposure to the grotesque, particularly intrusive imagery, contributes significantly to the development of psychiatric symptoms in war veterans (Green et al. 1989; Laufer et al. 1985a; Lifton 1973).

The study of exposure to grotesque death in war is difficult because of war's concurrent stressors; many of these stressors are unique to war. Ursano and McCarroll (1994) described deaths from "friendly fire," aspects of enemy dead, the deaths of women in combat, accidental deaths, and deaths from suicide. Friendly fire deaths usually are caused by accidents or errors by comrades in arms, although there are rare occasions when completion of a mission requires sacrificing one's own troops. Although such deaths may be considered avoidable and doubly tragic, the fallen are still regarded as comrades who gave their lives in the cause of war; such incidents usually are classified as combat deaths.

Dehumanizing the enemy is typical in war; at times, it has been part of the politics of war. Combat soldiers usually have few negative feelings about dead enemy soldiers unless they are humanized in some way that makes them appear to be like themselves. This humanizing process often occurs when a combat soldier uncovers an enemy soldier's personal effects, such as family pictures.

The deaths of military women in combat are still considered "unnatural"; women are not supposed to die in combat. Remains handlers often take special precautions with women's bodies that they do not take with those of men, such as keeping them covered and having a female chaperon with them while waiting and during autopsy.

Accidental deaths, such as those from vehicular mishaps or handling unexploded ordnance, often seem to be unnecessary events that should have been avoided had the victims been more careful. Suicides, although not unique to combat, often raise questions and controversy; soldiers generally regard suicide less sympathetically than combat deaths because suicides are self-inflicted.

"In Vietnam, death was our constant companion" (Spilka et al. 1978). For individuals who have participated in combat, seen combat deaths, or killed enemy soldiers or civilians, encounters with death may evoke complex feelings and reactions. Lifton (1973) noted two kinds of death that soldiers in Vietnam faced: those they witnessed and survived (such as the deaths of buddies) and those inflicted on the Vietnamese. Lifton (1973) characterized such memories of death witnessed or inflicted as the death imprint; witnessing subsequent deaths may activate that imprint.

Spilka et al. (1978) studied the death-related experiences of combat veterans before and during combat in Vietnam. Many soldiers spoke of death as a constant companion in Vietnam; the sight of American and enemy bodies was central to that experience. These investigators reported that 85% of the veterans they studied ($N = 104$) were present when someone they knew died. Approximately 86% of the veterans experienced extreme discomfort—to the point of sickness—when they saw an American body for the first time. The first sight of an enemy body, however, was associated with a significantly lower frequency of distress (64%). The researchers also found desensitization to the sight of remains: 76% of the subjects reported great upset at seeing an American body for the last time; the value reported for seeing the last enemy body was 39%. Reactivity was negatively correlated ($r = -.29$) with combat time.

The best predictors of distress related to the first viewing of a dead American soldier were having little or no prior contact with death, having children, low educational achievement, and thinking a lot about death when young. The more a veteran was bothered by the initial sight of an American body, the more he thought about being killed or wounded in Vietnam. Early experience with death was negatively correlated with distress on seeing the first dead American, fewer fears of one's own death, low expectations of becoming disabled from combat, and placing less value on one's life as a function of combat experience. The investigators concluded that this last negative association may reflect denial as a means of coping with the possibility of the person's own death; in other words, soldiers simply may not express their death fears. Denial also may explain why 38% of the veterans reported having no reaction and 33% felt no pain on being present when their buddies died.

Fontana et al. (1992) studied the combined contributions of objective characteristics of war zone stressors and the subjective meaning of those stressors. Their sample consisted of more than 1,700 treatment-seeking nonhospitalized veterans. One stressor was being an observer of killing; this stressor involved any of three elements: horror at witnessing atrocities or the results of atrocities, horror at exposure to the death and dismemberment of others, and horror at the continual stream of human remains to be processed. Observation of these traumas contributed significantly to hyperarousal, intrusion, numbing, and psychiatric distress—but not to a diagnosis of PTSD.

The Persian Gulf War and the invasion of Panama.   The United States sent soldiers into combat in two recent engagements: the 1989 invasion of Panama (Operation Just Cause) and the 1991 Persian Gulf War (Operation Desert Storm). For both of these operations, interviews and questionnaires were conducted with combat soldiers who handled the remains of American soldiers and civilians who had been killed and with professional remains handlers at the Dover Air Force Base mortuary (McCarroll et al. 1995). During Operation Just Cause, combat soldiers were exposed to and had to recover the bodies of civilians as well as their comrades; a control group consisted of soldiers who served in the same conflict but did not handle any remains.

Investigators examined incidents of remains handling by asking soldiers if they performed any of 13 different remains handling scenarios. These 13 scenarios varied with regard to the condition of the remains (e.g., mutilated or burned); the nature of the situation in which the remains were recovered including personal threat to the remains handler (e.g., under hostile fire or a booby-trapped body); and the soldier's relationship to the remains (e.g., body of a friend or a child). Soldiers were asked to rate the stress they felt at the time on a scale of 0 to 4, where 0 represented no stress and 4 was the highest they could imagine. When investigators compared the soldiers who responded positively to at least one of these 13 scenarios with those who responded negatively, the intrusion, avoidance, and total IES scores of the remains handlers were significantly higher than those not so exposed (see Table 3–1).

Investigators compared persons who handled human remains at the mortuary for Operation Desert Storm with non-remains handlers on IES scores approximately 3–5 months after the conflict (McCarroll et al. 1993a). Remains handlers reported significantly higher levels of intrusive and avoidant symptoms than non-remains handlers, and inexperienced remains handlers had more symptoms than those who were experienced. Similar high levels were observed

Table 3–1. Total IES, intrusion, and avoidance in combat soldiers working with dead bodies versus not exposed during Operation Just Cause, December 1989

	Total IES		Intrusion		Avoidance	
	Exposed	Not exposed	Exposed	Not exposed	Exposed	Not exposed
Mean	28.6*	19.8	14.7*	10.2	13.8*	9.4
SD	19.2	16.2	9.9	8.7	10.3	8.5
n	341	600	348	637	344	622

Note. SD = standard deviation.
*$P < .001$

1 year later (McCarroll et al. 1995). Sutker et al. (1994a)—using the SCID for PTSD diagnosis—also found higher rates of PTSD and of anxiety, anger, and somatic complaints among remains handlers in the Persian Gulf War.

DISCUSSION

Exposure to grotesque death is associated with acute and chronic posttraumatic stress disorder (Green 1993; Green et al. 1989; Laufer et al. 1985b; Lifton 1973; McCarroll et al. 1993a; Sutker et al. 1994a; Ursano and McCarroll 1994). The role of cognitions (beliefs and attitudes) is an important factor in adaptation after a traumatic event. Individuals and groups attach meaning to traumatic experiences to integrate those experiences into what is familiar and accommodate the changes required. People need to reestablish feelings of trust, safety, and predictability in the world and establish continuity among the past, present, and future. The experience of traumatic death shatters the assumption of invulnerability (i.e., "It can't happen to me") (Janoff-Bulman 1985, 1992); creates feelings of identification with the victim (i.e., "It could have been me") (Ursano and Fullerton 1990); and brings about a search for meaning (i.e., "Why me?") (Feifel 1959; Lifton 1967).

Posttraumatic stress responses are determined by type of stressor, stressor severity, and individual biological, psychosocial, and cognitive factors. Disaster workers anticipate the stress of upcoming work and therefore may begin the job with a substantial stress burden. The distress associated with anticipation of working with grotesque death, for example, is higher in nonvolunteers and those with no previous experience (McCarroll et al. 1993b, 1993c, 1995). Waiting time is a frequent stressor among professional firefighters (Ersland et al. 1989). Considering exposure to human remains as a special category of toxic exposure may be heuristically useful; dimensions such as the type of agent, frequency, intensity, and duration of exposure are risk factors for posttraumatic stress (Bartone et al. 1989; Ursano and McCarroll 1994).

The extent and intensity of sensory properties of remains—such as visual grotesqueness, smell, and tactile qualities—are important aspects of the stressor. Exposure to traumatic death evokes anxiety, intrusive images of death and dismemberment, and imagined risk. Lifton's work with Hiroshima survivors (Lifton 1967) described the intense preoccupation with mental images of mass death witnessed by the survivors. In those who bear witness to traumatic death, the death image can be intense and frightening. We know far less, however, about responses in people who do not directly witness the traumatic death of a family member or close friend.

Ursano and McCarroll (1994) examined the processes that exacerbate and protect against the stress of exposure to grotesque death. Emotional involvement and identification with the victims and families is common in remains handlers (McCarroll et al. 1993b). Identification and feelings of "knowing" the dead appear to heighten the trauma of the experience. Working with the bodies of children, for example, frequently elicits thoughts such as, "It could have been my child." Working with personal effects is another powerful stimulus for identification and subsequent distress. Seeing pictures of the deceased and their families heightens the distress of working with the dead. Identification may serve to eliminate the unfamiliar and the unknown qualities of the dead—changing what is new and novel into something familiar and part of the past (Ursano and Fullerton 1990).

To cope with the stress of exposure to grotesque death, disaster workers and soldiers develop cognitive and behavioral distancing (avoidance) strategies such as denial. Instructing workers to avoid looking at the faces of the dead and refrain from learning their names helps to "dehumanize" the body. Teaching persons who are exposed to traumatic death to decrease their identification and emotional involvement with victims and families may be effective in preventing posttraumatic stress among these individuals.

CONCLUSION

Most people exposed to traumatic death do not develop psychiatric disorders. Gaining a better understanding of the determinants of adaptation and recovery following trauma and disaster remains a challenge. Further research on how posttraumatic stress symptoms and disorders develop is needed. Such information could be useful in the development of better preparation, training, supervision, and support, as well as intervention programs for persons who experience the trauma of intimate contact with death. Additional research also is needed on the contextual variables that surround each individual: demographics, social support, preventive measures, treatments undertaken (or not), and the effects of time on psychological status. Longitudinal studies, including some examination of experiences before the occurrence of a traumatic event, are essential in addressing some of these issues.

Although exposure to death is stressful to almost everyone, the associated intrusive and avoidant behaviors and cognitions are not necessarily evidence of a pathologic process. Also, disaster workers take pride in their contributions in the face of the difficult challenge of working with traumatic death (McCarroll et al. 1993d). Individuals who witness extensive death in combat have complex reactions that are less well understood. Among the challenges mental health professionals will encounter in treating patients with death-associated trauma is how to use the individual's experiences with death to move toward health and to increase the value of life. Additional research about this powerful stressor is needed to further describe the normal "metabolism" of traumatic events.

REFERENCES

Alexander DA, Wells A: Reactions of police officers to body-handling after a major disaster: a before and after comparison. Br J Psychiatry 159: 547–555, 1991

American Psychiatric Association: Diagnosis and Statistical Manual of Mental Disorders, 3rd Edition. Washington, DC, American Psychiatric Association, 1980

American Psychiatric Association: Diagnosis and Statistical Manual of Mental Disorders, 3rd Edition, Revised. Washington, DC: American Psychiatric Association, 1987

American Psychiatric Association: Diagnostic and Statistical Manual of Mental Disorders, 4th Edition. Washington, DC, American Psychiatric Association, 1994

Andreasen NC: Posttraumatic stress disorder, in Comprehensive Textbook of Psychiatry. Edited by Kaplan HI, Sadock BJ. Baltimore, MD, Williams & Wilkins, 1985, pp 916–924

Appel JW: Preventive psychiatry, in Medical Department, United States Army: Neuropsychiatry In World War II, Vol 1. Edited by Glass AL, Burnucci RJ. Washington, DC, Department of the Army, Office of the Surgeon General, 1966, pp 403–410

Bartone PT, Ursano RJ, Wright FM, et al: The impact of a military air disaster on the health of assistance workers: a prospective study. J Nerv Ment Dis 177:317–328, 1989

Baum A, Solomon SD, Ursano RJ, et al: Emergency/disaster studies: practical, conceptual, and methodological issues, in International Handbook of Traumatic Stress Syndromes. Edited by Wilson JP, Raphael B. New York, Plenum, 1993, pp 125–134

Bolin R: Disaster characteristics and psychosocial impacts, in Disasters and Mental Health: Selected Contemporary Perspectives. Edited by Sowder BJ. Rockville, MD, U.S. Department of Health and Human Services, 1985, pp 3–28

Breslau N, Davis GC: Post-traumatic stress disorder: the etiologic specificity of wartime stressors. Am J Psychiatry 144:578–583, 1987

Breslau N, Davis GC: Posttraumatic stress disorder in an urban population of young adults: risk factors for chronicity. Am J Psychiatry 149:671–675, 1992

Breslau N, Davis GC, Andreski P, et al: Traumatic events and posttraumatic stress disorder in an urban population of young adults. Arch Gen Psychiatry 48:216–222, 1991

Chodoff P: Late effects of the concentration camp syndrome. Arch Gen Psychiatry 8:323–333, 1963

Corenblum B, Taylor PJ: Mechanisms of control of prolactin release in response to apprehension stress and anesthesia-surgery stress. Fertil Steril 36:712–715, 1981

Davidson JRT, Fairbank JA: The epidemiology of posttraumatic stress disorder, in Posttraumatic Stress Disorder: DSM-IV and Beyond. Edited by Davidson JRT, Foa EB. Washington, DC, American Psychiatric Press, 1993, pp 147–169

Davidson JRT, Foa EB (eds): Posttraumatic Stress Disorder: DSM-IV and Beyond. Washington, DC, American Psychiatric Press, 1993

Davidson J, Smith R: Traumatic experiences in psychiatric outpatients. J Trauma Stress 3:459–475, 1990

Demos GT, Hale HB, Williams EW: Anticipatory stress and flight stress in F-102 pilots. Aerosp Med 40:385–388, 1969

Derogatis LR: SCL-90-R Manual II. Towson, MD, Clinical Psychometric Research, 1983

Derogatis LR, Melisaratos N: The Brief Symptom Inventory: an introductory report. Psychol Med 13:595–605, 1983

Ersland S, Weisaeth L, Sund A: The stress upon rescuers involved in an oil rig disaster: Alexander L. Kielland 1980. Acta Psychiatr Scand 355:38–49, 1989

Etinger L, Strom A: Mortality and Morbidity After Excessive Stress. New York, Humanities Press, 1973

Feifel H: The Meaning of Death. New York, McGraw-Hill, 1959

Fenz WD, Epstein S: Gradients of physiological arousal in parachutists as a function of an approaching jump. Psychosom Med 29:33–51, 1967

Fontana A, Rosenheck R, Brett E: War zone traumas and posttraumatic stress disorder symptomatology. J Nerv Ment Dis 180:748–755, 1992

Foy D, Sipprelle R, Ruger D, et al: Etiology of post-traumatic stress disorder in Vietnam veterans: analysis of premilitary, military and combat exposure influences. J Consult Clin Psychol 52:79–87, 1984

Fullerton CS, McCarroll JE, Ursano RJ, et al: Psychological responses of rescue workers: fire fighters and trauma. Am J Orthopsychiatry 62: 371–378, 1992

Green BL: Defining trauma: terminology and generic stressor dimensions. Journal of Applied Social Psychology 20:1632–1642, 1990

Green BL: Identifying survivors at risk: trauma and stressors across events, in International Handbook of Traumatic Stress Syndromes. Edited by Wilson JP, Raphael B. New York, Plenum, 1993, pp 135–144

Green BL: Psychosocial research in traumatic stress: an update. J Trauma Stress 7:341–362, 1994

Green BL, Grace MC, Lindy JD, et al: Levels of functional impairment following a civilian disaster: the Beverly Hills Supper Club fire. J Consult Clin Psychol 5):573–580, 1983

Green BL, Lindy JD, Grace MC, et al: Multiple diagnosis in posttraumatic stress disorder: the role of war stressors. J Nerv Ment Dis 177:329–335, 1989

Green BL, Lindy JD, Grace MC, et al: Buffalo Creek survivors in the second decade: stability of stress symptoms. Am J Orthopsychiatry 20:43–54, 1990a

Green BL, Grace MC, Lindy JD, et al: Risk factors for PTSD and other diagnoses in the general sample of Vietnam Veterans. Am J Psychiatry 147:729–733, 1990b

Green BL, Lindy JD, Grace MC, et al: Chronic post-traumatic stress disorder and diagnostic comorbidity in a disaster sample. J Nerv Ment Dis 180:760–766, 1992

Grinker RR, Spiegel JJ: Men Under Stress. New York, McGraw-Hill, 1945

Gunderson JG, Sabo AN: The phenomenological and conceptual interface between borderline personality disorder and PTSD. Am J Psychiatry 150:19–27, 1993

Helzer JE, Robins LN: The Diagnostic Interview Schedule: its development, evolution, and use. Social Psychiatry Psychiatr Epidemiol 23:6–16, 1988

Helzer JE, Robins LN, McEvoy L: Post-traumatic stress disorder in the general population. N Engl J Med 317:1630–1634, 1987

Hershiser MR, Quarentelli EL: The handling of the dead in a disaster. Omega 7:195–203, 1976

Holen A: The North Sea oil rig disaster, in International Handbook of Traumatic Stress Syndromes. Edited by Wilson JP, Raphael B. New York, Plenum, 1993, pp 471–478

Horowitz M, Wilner N, Alvarez W: Impact of event scale: a measure of subjective stress. Psychosom Med 41:209–218, 1979

Horowitz MJ, Weiss DS, Marmor C: Commentary: diagnosis of posttraumatic stress disorder. J Nerv Ment Dis 175:267–268, 1987

Janoff-Bulman R: The aftermath of victimization: rebuilding shattered assumptions, in Trauma and its Wake: The Study and Treatment of Post-Traumatic Stress Disorder. Edited by Figley CR. New York, Brunner/Mazel, 1985, pp 15–35

Janoff-Bulman R: Shattered Assumptions: Towards a New Psychology of Trauma. New York, Free Press, 1992

Jones DR: Secondary disaster victims: the emotional effects of recovering and identifying human remains. Am J Psychiatry 142:303–307, 1985

Karam EG: The Lebanon wars: more data. Paper presented at the annual meeting of the International Traumatic Stress Society, Washington, DC, October 1991

Keane TM, Wolfe J: Comorbidity in post-traumatic stress disorder: an analysis of community and clinical studies. J Appl Soc Psychol 20:1776–1788, 1990

Kilpatrick DG, Resnick HS: Posttraumatic stress disorder associated with exposure to criminal victimization in clinical and community populations, in Posttraumatic Stress Disorder: DSM-IV and Beyond. Edited by Davidson JRT, Foa EB. Washington, DC, American Psychiatric Press, 1993, pp 113–143

Kilpatrick DG, Saunders BE, Veronen LJ, et al: Criminal victimization: lifetime prevalence, reporting to police, and psychological impact. Crime and Delinquency 33:479–489, 1987

Kilpatrick DG, Resnick HS, Amick A: Family members of homicide victims: search for meaning and post-traumatic stress disorder. Paper presented at the 97th annual convention of the American Psychological Association, New Orleans, LA, August 1989

Kilpatrick DG, Amick A, Resnick HS: The impact of homicide on surviving family members. Final Report, National Institute of Justice, Grant No. 87-IJ-CX-0017, 1990

Krystal H: Massive Psychic Trauma. New York, International Universities Press, 1968

Kulka RA, Schlenger WE: Survey research and field designs for the study of posttraumatic stress disorder, in International Handbook of Traumatic Stress Syndromes. Edited by Wilson JP, Raphael B. New York, Plenum, 1993, pp 145–157

Kulka RA, Schlenger WE, Fairbank JA, et al: Trauma and the Vietnam War Generation. New York, Brunner/Mazel, 1990

Kulka RA, Schlenger WE, Fairbank JA, et al: Assessment of posttraumatic stress disorder in the community: prospects and pitfalls from recent studies of Vietnam veterans. Psychological Assessment: A Journal of Consulting and Clinical Psychology 3:547–560, 1991

Laufer RS, Brett E, Gallops MS: Dimensions of posttraumatic stress disorder among Vietnam veterans. J Nerv Ment Dis 173:538–545, 1985a

Laufer RS, Brett E, Gallops MS: Symptom patterns associated with posttraumatic stress disorder among Vietnam veterans exposed to war trauma. Am J Psychiatry 142:1304–1311, 1985b

Lee KA, Vaillant GE, Torrey WC, et al: A 50-year prospective study of the psychological sequelae of World War II combat. Am J Psychiatry 152:516–522, 1995

Lifton RJ: Death in Life: Survivors of Hiroshima. London, Widenfeld and Nicolson, 1967

Lifton RJ: Home from the War. London, Wildwood House, 1973

Lindy JD, Green BL, Grace MC: Commentary: the stressor criterion. J Nerv Ment Dis 175:269–272, 1987

March JS: What constitutes a stressor? The "criterion A" issue, in Posttraumatic Stress Disorder: DSM-IV and Beyond. Edited by Davidson JRT, Foa EB. Washington, DC, American Psychiatric Press, 1993, pp 37–54

McCarroll JE, Fullerton CS, Ursano RJ: Stress of forensic dental identification: Branch Davidian disaster, Waco, TX. Paper presented at the International Society for Traumatic Stress Studies, Chicago, IL, November 1994

McCarroll JE, Ursano RJ, Fullerton CS: Posttraumatic stress disorder symptoms following recovery of war dead. Am J Psychiatry 150:1875–1877, 1993a

McCarroll JE, Ursano RJ, Fullerton CS, et al: Traumatic stress of a wartime mortuary: anticipation of mass death. J Nerv Ment Dis 181:545–551, 1993b

McCarroll JE, Ursano RJ, Ventis WL, et al: Anticipation of handling the dead: effects of gender and experience. Br J Clin Psychol 32:466–468, 1993c

McCarroll JE, Ursano RJ, Wright KM, et al: Handling of bodies after violent death: strategies for coping. Am J Orthopsychiatry 63:209–214, 1993d

McCarroll JE, Ursano RJ, Fullerton CS, et al: Gruesomeness, emotional attachment, and personal threat: dimensions of the anticipated stress of body recovery. J Trauma Stress 8:343–349, 1995

McCaughey BG, Hoffman KJ, Llewellyn CH: The human experience of earthquakes, in Individual and Community Responses to Trauma and Disaster: The Structure of Human Chaos. Edited by Ursano RJ, McCaughey BG, Fullerton CS. London, Cambridge University Press, 1994, pp 136–153

McFarlane AC: PTSD: synthesis of research and clinical studies: the Australia bushfire disaster, in International Handbook of Traumatic Stress Syndromes. Edited by Wilson JP, Raphael B. New York, Plenum, 1993, pp 421–430

Mefferd BR, Wieland BA: Comparison of responses to anticipated stress and stress. Psychosom Med 28:795–807, 1966

Meichenbaum D: Cognitive-Behavior Modification. New York, Plenum, 1977

Norris F: Epidemiology of trauma: frequency and impact of different potentially traumatic events on different demographic groups. J Consult Clin Psychol 60:409–418, 1992

Paton D: Disaster relief work: an assessment of training effectiveness. J Trauma Stress 7:275–288, 1994

Penzien DB, Hursey KG, Kotses H, et al: The effects of anticipatory stress on heart rate and T-wave amplitude. Biol Psychiatry 15:241–248, 1982

Raphael B: When Disaster Strikes. New York, Basic Books, 1986

Resnick HS, Kilpatrick DG, Dansky BS, et al: Prevalence of civilian trauma and posttraumatic stress disorder in a representative national sample of women. J Consult Clin Psychol 61:984–991, 1993

Rundell JR, Ursano RJ, Holloway HC, et al: Psychiatric responses to trauma. Hosp Comm Psychiatry 40:68–74, 1989

Shore JH, Tatum EL, Vollmer WM: Psychiatric reactions to disaster: the Mount St. Helen's experience. Am J Psychiatry 143:590–595, 1986

Short P: Victims and helpers, in Natural Hazards in Australia. Edited by Heathcote RL, Tong BG. Canberra, Australian Academy of Science, 1979, pp 112–130

Smith E, North C: Posttraumatic stress disorder in natural disasters and technological accidents, in International Handbook of Traumatic Stress Syndromes. Edited by Wilson JP, Raphael B. New York, Plenum, 1993, pp 405–420

Solomon SD, Canino GJ: Appropriateness of DSM-III-R criteria of post-traumatic stress disorder. Compr Psychiatry 31:227–237, 1990

Spiegel D, Cardeña E: Disintegrated experience: the dissociative disorders revisited. J Abnorm Psychol 100:366–378, 1991

Spilka B, Friedman L, Rosenberg D: Death and Vietnam: some combat veteran experiences and perspectives, in Stress Disorders Among Vietnam Veterans. Edited by Figley CR. New York, Brunner/Mazel, 1978

Spitzer R, Williams J, Gibbon M: Structured Clinical Interview for DSM-III-R, Version NP-V. New York, New York State Psychiatric Institute, Biometrics Research Department, 1987

Steinglass P, Gerrity E: Natural disasters and post-traumatic stress disorder: short-term versus long-term recovery in two disaster-affected communities. Journal of Applied Social Psychology 20:1746–1765, 1990

Sutker PB, Uddo M, Brailey K, et al: Psychological symptoms and psychiatric diagnoses in Operation Desert Storm troops serving graves registration duties. J Trauma Stress 7:159–171, 1994a

Sutker PB, Uddo M, Brailey K, et al: Psychopathology in war-zone deployed and non-deployed troops assigned graves registration duties. J Abnorm Psychol 103:383–390, 1994b

Taylor AJW, Frazer AG: The stress of post-disaster body handling and victim identification work. J Human Stress 8:4–12, 1982

Trimble M: Post-traumatic Neurosis. New York, Wiley, 1981

Ursano RJ: Commentary: post-traumatic stress disorder: the stressor criterion. J Nerv Ment Dis 75:273–275, 1987

Ursano RJ, Fullerton CS: Cognitive and behavioral responses to trauma. J Appl Psychol 20:1766–1775, 1990

Ursano RJ, McCarroll JE: The nature of the traumatic stressor: handling dead bodies. J Nerv Ment Dis 178:396–398, 1990

Ursano RJ, McCarroll JE: Exposure to traumatic death: the nature of the stressor, in Individual and Community Responses to Trauma and Disaster: The Structure of Human Chaos. Edited by Ursano RJ, McCaughey BG, Fullerton CS. London, Cambridge University Press, 1994, pp 46–71

Ursano RJ, Boydstun JA, Wheatley RD: Psychiatric illness in U.S. Air Force Vietnam prisoners of war: a five-year follow-up. Am J Psychiatry 138:310–314, 1981

Ursano RJ, McCaughey BC, Fullerton CS: Individual and Community Responses to Trauma and Disaster: The Structure of Human Chaos. London, Cambridge University Press, 1994

Ursano RJ, Fullerton CS, Kao T-C, et al: Longitudinal assessment of posttraumatic stress disorder and depression after exposure to traumatic death. J Nerv Ment Dis 183:36–42, 1995

Weisæth L, Eitinger L: Posttraumatic stress phenomena: common themes across wars, disasters, and traumatic events, in International Handbook of Traumatic Stress Syndromes. Edited by Wilson JP, Raphael B. New York, Plenum, 1993, pp 69–77

Weiss DS: Structured clinical interview techniques, in International Handbook of Traumatic Stress Syndromes. Edited by Wilson JP, Raphael B. New York, Plenum, 1993, pp 179–180

Wilson JP, Raphael B (eds): International Handbook of Traumatic Stress Syndromes. New York, Plenum, 1993

Wolfe J, Keane TM: New perspectives in the assessment and diagnosis of combat-related posttraumatic stress disorder, in International Handbook of Traumatic Stress Syndromes. Edited by Wilson JP, Raphael B. New York, Plenum, 1993, pp 167–177

Zung WWK: A self-rating depression scale. Arch Gen Psychiatry 12:63–70, 1965

Chapter 4

Posttraumatic Responses in Spouse/Significant Others of Disaster Workers

Carol S. Fullerton, Ph.D., and Robert J. Ursano, M.D.

Over the past decade, a plethora of investigators have conducted research on trauma and disaster (see Davidson and Foa 1993; Green and Lindy 1994; Ursano et al. 1994; Wilson and Raphael 1993). Most of this research relates to individuals who are direct victims of traumatic events. Psychiatrists increasingly recognize, however, that disasters and other traumatic events also have psychiatric consequences for individuals other than the primary victims; such nonvictims also may develop psychiatric illness.

DSM-IV (American Psychiatric Association 1994) now defines bearing witness to a trauma or being confronted by the traumatic experience of a family member or close friend as a significant stressor with potential psychiatric consequences (criterion A for posttraumatic stress disorder [PTSD] and acute stress disorder). Psychiatrists know much less about this type of exposure than they do about direct exposure, however. In particular, we know very little about the mechanisms of transmission of posttraumatic stress to persons who witness or learn about the traumatic exposure of a significant other (as opposed to those who are directly exposed and suffer personal life threat).

In this chapter, we describe a study of one group of individuals who fit this indirect exposure category of acute posttraumatic stress: spouses/significant others (SSOs) of disaster workers after a mass-casualty airplane crash. We compared this group with two matched control groups. The SSOs were not directly exposed to the trauma but had exposure to partners who performed disaster work at the crash site. Our preliminary data are directed at answering five questions:

• Do the SSOs of disaster workers provide support?
• Do the SSOs of disaster workers receive support from family and friends?
• Do the SSOs of disaster workers experience psychological and physiological stress?
• Is providing support associated with psychological distress in the SSOs of disaster workers?
• Is the stress of a disaster worker's SSO associated with the stress of the disaster worker?

BEARING WITNESS TO TRAUMA AND PROVIDING SUPPORT: PSYCHIATRIC CONSEQUENCES IN SPOUSES/SIGNIFICANT OTHERS

Two bodies of literature suggest the possibility of stress effects in family members of primary victims of trauma. The literature on PTSD suggests an association between witnessing or learning of the traumatic experience of a family member and the development of PTSD. The literature on psychosocial support suggests that providing support to family members exposed to trauma is stressful and has psychological and physical health consequences.

Posttraumatic Stress Disorder

Although PTSD usually is associated with primary exposure to trauma, family members of trauma victims also may develop PTSD and related symptoms. The DSM-III-R (American Psychiatric Association 1987) stressor criterion for PTSD included ". . . a serious threat or harm to one's children, spouse, or other close relatives and friends" (p. 250). The DSM-IV (American Psychiatric Association 1994) stressor criterion includes ". . . Events experienced by others that are learned about [such as] . . . violent personal assault, serious accident, or serious injury experienced by a family member or a close friend; learning about the sudden unexpected death of a family member or close friend . . ." (p. 424). Thus, the psychiatric profession recognizes that family members of victims and disaster workers who are at risk of injury are potential traumatic stress victims.

Support Provision

In addition to symptoms of PTSD that may result from hearing about a family member's traumatic experience, individuals may be subject to other characteristic symptoms because of their role as support providers (one of the potential stressors inherent in disaster worker SSOs). Investigators have developed a body of research relating to this phenomenon, although a detailed review is beyond the scope of this chapter. For a general review, see Biegel et al. (1991); for a review specific to emotional disturbance in the family, see Brody and Sigel (1990).

A substantial body of research documents the beneficial health effects of receiving psychosocial support from spouses, other family members, and friends at times of stress (see Cohen and Wills 1985; House et al. 1988). These beneficial effects also appear after large-scale traumatic events (e.g., Green et al. 1985; S. D. Solomon et al. 1989). Providing support to family members can be stressful for the support provider, however, and strain the family unit—particularly after traumatic event exposure (Fullerton et al. 1993; Shumaker and Brownell 1984; S. D. Solomon et al. 1987; Taylor 1990). Although women may be more likely than men to respond supportively during times of stress (Kessler and McLeod 1985), women also may experience strong social supports as burdensome during these times (S. D. Solomon et al. 1987).

Psychiatric effects of support provision. Symptoms associated with the stress of familial support provision include depression, hostility, and anxiety. Many studies have reported elevated rates of depression among support providers, compared with age- and gender-matched persons not providing support (e.g., Gallagher et al. 1989; Kiecolt-Glaser et al. 1987; Pruncho and Potashnik 1989; Stoller and Pugliesi 1989). The more impaired the patient, the greater the depressive symptomatology in the support provider; female support providers tend to be more depressed than male support providers.

Using the Brief Symptom Inventory (BSI) (Derogatis and Spencer 1982) to assess psychiatric symptoms in support providers for dementia patients, Anthony-Bergstone et al. (1988) found elevated levels of hostility, compared with population norms, in male and female support providers who were young adults or at least 60 years old (versus those who were middle-aged). High levels of anxiety followed a similar age pattern in the female support providers but not in the men providing support; the researchers found high levels of depression only in older female support providers (Anthony-Bergstone et al. 1988). Using the Minnesota Multiphasic Personality Inventory (MMPI) (Hathaway and McKinley 1989), Fitting et al. (1986) also found higher rates of depression in female support providers for dementia patients than male support providers.

In a study of wives of combat veterans suffering from combat stress reaction and PTSD, Z. Solomon et al. (1991) reported increased somatic complaints and psychiatric distress among the wives. These investigators suggested that stress in the wife was associated with the increased responsibility secondary to the husband's illness, as well as identification with the husband's symptoms.

Physical health.   Providing support also is associated with poorer self-reported physical health. Haley et al. (1987) found that support providers reported poorer overall health and more chronic illness than a group of matched non-support providers. In a survey of 678 elderly people, Satariano et al. (1984) found that one spouse's ill health was a strong predictor of poor health in the other spouse. The mechanisms that propagate poor health in support providers are unclear; they may include the stress of support provision itself, empathy, and shared environmental exposure.

Studies of health care utilization in support providers have produced conflicting results. Although some researchers have found that support providers report more frequent physician visits and more frequent use of prescription drugs than do non-support providers (Haley et al. 1987), other investigators have reported no differences in support providers' use of medical services (Kiecolt-Glaser et al. 1987). Several studies have reported high rates of psychotropic drug use in support providers (e.g., Clipp and George 1990; George and Gwyther 1986).

Providing support itself may entail demands that limit the opportunity to use health care and cause changes in health behaviors. Pennebaker and colleagues (Pennebaker et al. 1988) found a relationship between disclosure of traumatic events, fewer health center visits, and decreased autonomic arousal. They suggested that couple relationships and communication patterns may affect health care utilization and health outcomes.

PSYCHOSOCIAL RESPONSES IN SPOUSES/
SIGNIFICANT OTHERS OF DISASTER WORKERS
FOLLOWING A PLANE CRASH:
A PRELIMINARY REPORT

We conducted a preliminary investigation of acute posttraumatic stress in SSOs of disaster workers after a mass-casualty airplane crash, as well as in two matched control groups. The SSOs were not directly exposed to the trauma but had exposure to partners who performed disaster work at the crash site. In this section, we describe the support provided by disaster worker SSOs, the distress in these SSOs, and preliminary data on the relationship between distress in the SSO and distress in the disaster worker. (We are currently analyzing the longitudinal data and additional comparisons, which we will report elsewhere.)

The Disaster

On July 19, 1989, a United Airlines DC-10 carrying 296 passengers and crew crash-landed at Sioux City, Iowa, following a midair malfunction that caused complete failure of the plane's hydraulic system. Casualties included 112 people who died. Rescue personnel were alerted approximately a $1/2$ hour before the attempted landing, which occurred on an unused runway at the Sioux Gateway Airport; they awaited the attempted landing just off the runways. Upon touchdown, the plane broke apart and burst into flames, and the wreckage was scattered on and off the runway and in adjoining corn and soybean fields. Some victims, still in their seats, were thrown from the aircraft; others died in the burning fuselage. Of the 184 survivors, more than 70 literally walked away from the crash.

Consultation and Research Relating to the Disaster

Our research/consultation group initiated a longitudinal follow-up of the disaster workers and provided consultation to the community. One month after the disaster, we distributed 440 surveys to Sioux City Air National Guard disaster workers; 212 surveys were completed and returned by these disaster workers (48% return rate). Disaster workers also received surveys for their SSOs, if appropriate. Approximately 70% ($n = 148$) of the 212 disaster workers who completed the surveys were married, and 133 disaster worker SSOs completed and returned surveys (90% return rate).

Concurrently, we distributed surveys to two comparison groups: Sioux City Air National Guard members who did not participate in the disaster work for a variety of reasons (e.g., away at the time, could not get onto the base) and their SSOs and Air National Guard members (and SSOs) from Sioux Falls, South Dakota (a similar community 90 miles away, matched for socioeconomic level, geography, urban/rural location, and military unit/job). Of 750 Sioux City nonworkers, 102 agreed to participate and completed surveys. Of these 102 nonworkers, approximately 70% ($n = 71$) were married; 63 nonworker SSOs (89%) completed and returned surveys. A total of 428 members of the Sioux Falls Air National Guard unit—approximately 300 (70%) of whom were married—completed surveys, and 255 Sioux Falls Guard SSOs (85%) completed and returned surveys. The median completion date, 2 $1/2$ months after the disaster, did not differ across the study groups.

Assessments.   We measured demographic data, prior disaster experience, receiving and giving support, activities with SSO, stress on oneself and family members, medical care utilization, sleep patterns, fatigue immediately following the disaster, identification with disaster victims, and major life events. We used standardized and self-report measures to assess psychological symptomatology, coping, social support, and other variables.

Subjects.   Our preliminary study focused on disaster worker SSOs ($N = 135$) who completed the 1-month postdisaster questionnaire and the two matched SSO control groups—the nonworker SSOs ($N = 63$) and the Sioux Falls SSOs ($N = 255$). The SSO groups did not significantly differ on demographics (see Table 4–1) and rate of survey return. The majority of SSOs were married (most to enlisted men), white females in their late 30s (mean age = 38) with at least some college. The homogeneity of education and spouses' rank indicated that there were no differences in socioeconomic status, although the proportion of SSOs who were employed varied across the disaster worker SSOs, nonworker SSOs, and Sioux Falls SSOs: 61%, 50%, and 38%, respectively (χ^2 = (2) 18.995, P < .001).

Results

Support provided by SSOs. The majority of disaster worker SSOs (83.3%) reported providing support (see Table 4–2). This proportion was significantly higher than that for nonworker SSOs (42.6%) or Sioux Falls SSOs (63.2%) (χ^2 = 33.374 (2), P < .001).

Support received from family and friends. We assessed social support from family and friends separately using self-report Likert scales (1 = unsupportive, 2 = neutral, 3 = supportive). The majority of worker SSOs (83.1%) reported receiving support from family at the time of the disaster and the week that followed (Table 4–2). In the control groups, 73.9% of nonworker SSOs and 59.6% of the Sioux Falls SSOs reported receiving support from family. The overall chi square for the three SSO groups was significant (χ^2 = 28.704 (4), P < .001). Furthermore, 77.5% of the worker SSOs, 59.5% of the nonworker SSOs, and 48.9% of the Sioux Falls SSOs reported receiving support from friends (χ^2 = 23.948 (4), P < .001).

Intrusive and avoidant symptoms. We used the Impact of Event Scale (IES) (Horowitz et al. 1979b) to examine intrusive and avoidant symptoms in the worker SSOs during the first week after the disaster. Disaster worker SSOs had IES total scores of M = 25.20 (SD = 16.43) during the first week after the disaster; nonworker SSOs had total IES scores of M = 22.22 (SD = 15.90), and Sioux Falls SSOs had scores of M = 13.58 (SD = 13.09) (F = 30.20, [2,443], P < .0001). Based on IES thresholds identified by Horowitz et al. (1979b)—which assign levels of clinical concern: low = ≤8.5, medium = 8.6–19.0, and high > 19.0— 59.5% of the disaster worker SSOs scored in the high range of clinical concern compared with 47.6% of the nonworker SSOs and 26.6% of the Sioux Falls SSOs (χ^2 = 51.741 (4), P < .001). These results compare with IES scores reported by Steinglass and Gerrity (1990) for two disaster community samples; they found that at 4 months, 76% of the population of a community struck by a tornado and 49%

Table 4–1.   Demographics of disaster worker SSOs, nonworker SSOs, and Sioux Falls SSOs

	Disaster worker SSOs (N = 133)		Nonworker SSOs (N = 63) (control subjects)		Sioux Falls SSOs (N = 255) (control subjects)	
	N	%	N	%	N	%
Sex						
Male	3	2	7	11	14	6
Female	130	98	56	89	241	94
Race						
White	132	99	63	100	252	99
Nonwhite	1	1	0	0	3	1
Marital status						
Married	124	93	57	90	237	93
Single	9	7	6	10	18	7
Education						
High school	50	37	31	50	81	32
Some college	57	43	20	31	128	50
College degree ≥	26	20	12	19	46	18
Employed*						
Yes	81	61	32	51	97	38
No	52	39	31	49	158	62
Rank of partner						
Officer	27	20	9	14	46	18
Enlisted	106	80	54	86	209	82

Note.   SSO = spouses/significant others. Figures may not sum to 100% because of rounding. The ages of subjects were as follows (means ± standard deviation): disaster worker SSOs: 37.73 ± 9.33; nonworker SSOs: 35.68 ± 8.72; Sioux Falls SSOs: 37.10 ± 9.41.
*$P < .001$

of a community struck by a flood scored in the high clinical concern group on the IES.

Self-reported stress.   We assessed self-reported stress during the first week after the crash on a Likert scale from 1 to 7 (1 = none,

Table 4–2. Providing support and receiving support from family and friends

	Disaster worker SSOs		Nonworker SSOs (control subjects)		Sioux Falls SSOs (control subjects)	
	N	%	N	%	N	%
Providing support*	110	83.3	26	42.6	67	63.2
Receiving support from						
Family**	98	83.1	34	73.9	87	59.6
Friends***	86	77.4	25	59.5	68	48.9

Note. SSO = spouses/significant others.
*χ^2 = 33.37(4), P < .001.   **χ^2 = 28.70(4), P < .001.   ***χ^2 = 23.95(4), P < .001

7 = high). Mean scores for worker SSOs, nonworker SSOs, and Sioux Falls SSOs were $\overline{X}$ = 3.88 (SD = 1.57), $\overline{X}$ = 3.68 (SD = 1.53), and $\overline{X}$ = 3.26 (SD = 1.49), respectively (F = 7.66, [2,435], P < .001). Multiple comparisons (Bonferonni corrected) indicated a significant difference between worker SSOs and Sioux Falls SSOs (P = .001); no other pairs differed significantly. The self-report measures were moderately to highly correlated with the total IES, intrusion, and avoidance scores.

Sleep, fatigue, and return to normal pace. Disaster worker SSOs reported a mean of 6.50 (SD = 1.24) hours of sleep during the week after the disaster. We assessed fatigue the day after the disaster on a Likert scale (0 = none, 7 = very); mean fatigue among disaster worker SSOs was moderate (X = 3.73, SD = 1.82). Among disaster worker SSOs, 19.1% reported that the subsidence of symptoms of physiologic stress (e.g., "adrenalin stopped pumping," "pace back to normal") took 1–2 days after the plane disaster, 21.4% reported symptom subsidence taking 3–4 days, 11.5% reported 5–6 days; 11.5% reported needing more than 1 week after the disaster to return to a normal pace. However, 36.6% reported no change in their normal pace after the disaster.

Health care utilization. We examined health care utilization to further assess behavioral measures of physical illness. We measured health care utilization by counting the number of people seeing physicians for annual physical checkups, physical problems, and emotional problems the previous 3 months. Among worker SSOs, 3.2% reported seeking help for emotional problems, 10.5% had annual physicals, and 16.9% saw a physician for physical problems.

Providing support and acute stress (IES).   Disaster worker SSOs who provided support had substantial levels of stress 1 week after the disaster. Disaster worker SSOs who provided support had higher total IES and higher levels of IES intrusive symptoms than disaster worker SSOs who did not provide support (total IES = 27.0 versus 18.8, IES intrusion = 15.7 versus 10.1, for support providers versus nonproviders, respectively; see Table 4–3). Avoidant symptoms did not differ significantly between support providers and nonproviders.

Anxiety and depression 2 months after the disaster.   Two months after the disaster, 26.7% of the disaster worker SSOs who reported providing support were at the 90th percentile of depression on the SCL-90-R (Derogatis 1983); 22.2% were at the 90th percentile for anxiety.

Acute IES in disaster worker SSOs compared with disaster workers (1 week after the disaster).   The disaster was significantly correlated with those for the disaster workers themselves ($r = .22$, $P = .02$). Further analyses indicated that the correlation was primarily related to intrusive symptoms—that is, the level of intrusive symptoms in SSOs was moderately correlated with the level of intrusive symptoms in disaster workers ($r = .27$, $P = .004$). Symptoms of avoidance in SSOs were not correlated with such symptoms in disaster workers.

DISCUSSION

Posttraumatic stress in familial support providers after acute trauma has not been well studied. As a consequence, the mechanisms of transmission of posttraumatic stress to familial support providers following acute trauma exposure of a family member are not well understood.

SSOs involved in our study provided substantial support to disaster workers and received support from family and friends. Disaster worker SSOs also reported substantial intrusive and avoidant symptoms and self-reported distress. They reported decreased sleep after the disaster, and many required several days to weeks to return to "normal." Disaster worker SSOs who reported providing support also reported substantial distress and more intrusive symptoms than SSOs who did not provide support. (Little can be said about health care utilization until comparisons can be made with the control groups.)

These findings suggest that exposure as a disaster worker SSO may be a risk factor for psychiatric distress after a disaster. This disaster, although sudden and unexpected, was not enduring and did not involve substantial separation or direct effects on the SSOs—as might be true in widespread natural disaster such as an earthquake. Thus, this sample of disaster worker SSOs represents nearly pure exposure to the disaster worker as the source of the SSOs' distress (i.e., without the confounding effects of other event-related exposure).

Several mechanisms may explain distress and potential illness in disaster worker SSOs: fear and anticipated loss secondary to a partner's trauma exposure; the demands of providing support itself; nonreciprocal support; recall of traumatic events in one's own past; limited attention to one's own needs for social support/support networks and health care utilization; poor health behaviors; identification with a partner's distress; repressed feelings of dissatisfaction or anger at the disaster worker; and experiencing the distress of others in the disaster community.

Posttraumatic Stress and Support Provision Among Disaster Worker SSOs

Even disaster workers are likely to be unprepared for a disaster of substantial magnitude; as a result, they may need increased support

Table 4–3. Support provision and acute stress (IES) among disaster worker spouses/significant others

| | Support provision | |
	Yes	No
Total IES*	27.0	18.8
Intrusion*	15.7	10.1
Avoidance	11.4	8.7

Note. *$P < .05$

from SSOs. The relationship between disaster workers' expectations of support and the actual support they receive may be important to subsequent expectations placed on the SSO (Kaniasty et al. 1990). These expectations may cause stress in the caregiver SSO and in the couple relationship. Moreover, the psychosocial support provided to disaster workers may not be reciprocated to SSOs. These factors may contribute to stress in SSO caregivers (Ingersoll-Dayton and Antonucci 1988). The exposure of disaster workers to threat and death may lead directly to SSO fear and concern about loss and the future. Thus, exposure to the disaster worker, the need to provide support to the disaster worker, and the vicarious exposure to the disaster may put the support provider at risk for posttraumatic symptoms.

Being close to someone exposed to a traumatic event can be a powerful reminder of earlier stressful or traumatic experiences in one's own life (Holloway and Ursano 1984). Lifton (1993) suggested that the patterns of a survivor's experience may lead persons close to the survivor to recall similar feelings from their own past (e.g., separation and threat). Furthermore, media coverage of large-scale disasters and recent warfare may be difficult to avoid. For many people, bearing vicarious witness to current traumatic events recalls or reconstructs past events in their own lives. Similarly, one mechanism of transmission of exposure to traumatic stress from disaster workers to their SSOs is the recall of past stressors.

Physical Health in Disaster Worker SSOs

Direct assessment of health care utilization, along with more common self-reports, can provide a more complete picture of health responses following trauma in disaster worker SSOs. Changes in health behaviors (e.g., diet, exercise, sleep, weight, smoking, alcohol) represent one mechanism by which stress can affect health (Coyne and Holroyd 1982; Wetzler and Ursano 1988). Langlie (1977) found that people with many demands on their time reported feeling a lack of control and perceived the costs of maintaining good health practices as high. This response may be particularly prevalent in support providers after a disaster.

People in high-stress conditions also commonly report increased alcohol consumption and smoking compared with those in low-stress conditions (Horowitz et al. 1979a; Schachter et al. 1977); this behavior may reflect a kind of self-medication. Findings from the Alameda County Study (Berkman and Breslow 1983; Wingard and Berkman 1985) indicated a positive association between social networks and health behaviors such as hours of sleep, drinking, smoking, physical exercise, and weight (see House et al. 1988). The demands of support provision may lead to decreases in social networks and thus effect health or health behaviors.

Another mechanism for disturbed health in disaster worker SSOs may be their own PTSD. In a 2-year follow-up of 51 rape victims, Waigandt et al. (1990) found significant differences between victims and matched control subjects in current illness symptoms (e.g., high or low blood pressure, severe colds, headaches, stomach pains) measured by the Cornell Medical Index Health Questionnaire (Brodman et al. 1949). Similarly, the relationship of PTSD and health in caregivers may be mediated by health behaviors.

Researchers have found a relationship between PTSD and poor health practices in veterans (Card 1987; Shalev et al. 1990) and in nonveteran community samples (Gleser et al. 1981; Helzer et al. 1987). Helzer et al. (1987) found that individuals with PTSD were more likely to abuse drugs and alcohol than other persons in the general population, and substance abuse is a common comorbid disorder in veteran populations with PTSD (Kulka et al. 1990). Shalev et al. (1990) reported increased cigarette use among individuals with PTSD; in a sample of Buffalo Creek disaster victims, Gleser et al. (1981) found a 44% increase in cigarette smoking and a 52% increase in the use of prescription drugs, along with significantly increased alcohol consumption.

CONCLUSIONS

Although none of the disaster worker SSOs in our study were direct victims of the plane crash—nor were they exposed to the disaster site—they nonetheless showed moderate levels of posttraumatic distress from their exposure via the disaster workers. Future research should examine SSOs to further elucidate the mechanisms or avenues of transmission of stress, altered health, and health behaviors in disaster worker SSOs. Such research will enable psychiatrists to identify SSOs at high risk of posttraumatic stress and altered health. The development of interventions to decrease distress in SSOs also would increase the support available to disaster workers. Involving SSOs in debriefing and education programs for disaster workers after a disaster event may be reasonable first interventions to accomplish these goals.

REFERENCES

American Psychiatric Association: Diagnostic and Statistical Manual of Mental Disorders, 3rd Edition, Revised. Washington, DC: American Psychiatric Association, 1987

American Psychiatric Association: Diagnostic and Statistical Manual of Mental Disorders, 4th Edition. Washington, DC, American Psychiatric Association, 1994

Anthony-Bergstone CR, Zarit SH, Gatz M: Symptoms of psychological distress among caregivers of dementia patients. Psychol Aging 3:245–248, 1988

Berkman LF, Breslow L: Health practices and mortality risk, in Health and Ways of Living. Edited by Berkman L, Breslow L. New York, Oxford University Press, 1983, pp 113–160

Biegel DE, Sales E, Schulz R: Family Caregiving in Chronic Illness: Alzheimer's Disease, Cancer, Heart Disease, Mental Illness, and Stroke. Newbury Park, CA, Sage, 1991

Brodman K, Erdmann AJ, Lorge I, et al: The Cornell Medical Index. JAMA 140:530, 1949

Brody GH, Sigel IE (eds): Methods of Family Research: Biographies of Research Projects, Vol 2: Clinical Populations. Hillsdale, NJ, Erlbaum, 1990

Card JJ: Epidemiology of PTSD in a national cohort of Vietnam veterans. J Clin Psychol 43:6–17, 1987

Clipp EC, George LK: Psychotropic drug use among caregivers of patients with dementia. J Am Geriatr Soc 38:227–235, 1990

Cohen S, Wills TA: Stress, social support, and the buffering hypothesis. Psychol Bull 98:310–357, 1985

Coyne JC, Holroyd K: Stress, coping, and illness: a transactional perspective, in Handbook of Clinical Health Psychology. Edited by Millon T, Green C, Meagher R. New York, Plenum, 1982, pp 103–127

Davidson JRT, Foa EB (eds): Posttraumatic Stress Disorder: DSM-IV and Beyond. Washington, DC, American Psychiatric Press, 1993

Derogatis LR: SCL-90-R Manual II. Towson, MD, Clinical Psychometric Research, 1983

Derogatis LP, Spencer MS: The Brief Symptom Inventory (BSI): Administration, Scoring, and Procedures Manual. Baltimore, MD, Clinical Psychometric Research, 1982

Fitting M, Rabins P, Lucas MJ, et al: Caregivers of dementia patients: a comparison of husbands and wives. Gerontologist 26:248–252, 1986

Fullerton CS, Wright K, Ursano, RJ: Social support of disaster workers: the role of significant others. Nordic Journal of Psychiatry 47:315–324, 1993

Gallagher D, Rose J, Rivera P, et al: Prevalence of depression in family caregivers. Gerontologist 29:449–456, 1989

George LK, Gwyther LP: Caregiver well-being: a multidimensional examination of family caregivers of demented adults. Gerontologist 26: 253–259, 1986

Gleser GC, Green BL, Winget CN: Prolonged Psychosocial Effects of Disaster: A Study of Buffalo Creek. New York, Academic Press, 1981

Green BL, Lindy JD: Post-traumatic stress disorder in victims of disasters. Psychiatr Clin North Am 17:301–309, 1994

Green BL, Grace MC, Gleser GC: Identifying survivors at risk: long-term impairment following the Beverly Hills Supper Club fire. J Consult Clin Psychol 53:672–678, 1985

Haley WE, Levine EG, Brown SL, et al: Stress, appraisal, coping, and social support as predictors of adaptational outcome among dementia caregivers. Psychol Aging 2:323–330, 1987

Hathaway SR, McKinley JC: Minnesota Multiphasic Personality Inventory—2. Minneapolis, University of Minnesota, 1989

Helzer JE, Robins LN, McEvoy L: Post-traumatic stress disorder in the general population. N Engl J Med 317:1630–1634, 1987

Holloway HC, Ursano RJ: The Vietnam veteran: memory, social context, and metaphor. Psychiatry 47:103–108, 1984

Horowitz MJ, Benfari R, Hulley S, et al: Life events, risk factors, and coronary disease. Psychosomatics 20:586–592, 1979a

Horowitz M, Wilner N, Alvarez W: Impact of Event Scale: a measure of subjective stress. Psychosom Med 41:209–218, 1979b

House JS, Landis KR, Umberson, D: Social relationships and health. Science 241:540–545, 1988

Ingersoll-Dayton B, Antonucci TC: Reciprocal and nonreciprocal social support: contrasting sides of intimate relationships. J Gerontol 43: 65–73, 1988

Kaniasty K, Norris F, Murrell SA: Received and perceived social support following natural disaster. J Applied Soc Psychol 20:85–114, 1990

Kessler RC, McLeod JD: Social support and mental health in community samples, in Social Support and Health. Edited by Cohen S, Syme SL. New York, Academic Press, 1985, pp 219–240

Kiecolt-Glaser JK, Glaser R, Shuttleworth EE, et al: Chronic stress and immunity in family caregivers of Alzheimer's disease patients. Psychosom Med 49:523–535, 1987

Kulka RA, Schlenger WE, Fairbank JA, et al: Trauma and the Vietnam War Generation. New York, Brunner/Mazel, 1990

Langlie JK: Social networks, health beliefs, and preventive health behavior. J Health Soc Behav 18:244–260, 1977

Lifton RJ: The Protean Self: Human Resilience in an Age of Fragmentation. New York, Basic Books, 1993

Pennebaker JW, Kiecolt-Glaser JK, Glaser R: Disclosure of traumas and immune function: health implications for psychotherapy. J Consult Clin Psychol 56:239–245, 1988

Pruncho RA, Potashnik SL: Caregiving spouses: physical and mental health in perspective. J Am Geriatr Soc 37:697-705, 1989

Satariano W, Minkler MA, Langhauser C: The significance of an ill spouse for assessing health differences in an elderly population. J Am Geriatr Soc 32:187–190, 1984

Schachter S, Silverstein B, Kozlowski LT, et al: Effects of stress on cigarette smoking and urinary pH. J Exp Psychol Gen 106:24–30, 1977

Shalev A, Bleich A, Ursano, RJ: Posttraumatic stress disorder: somatic comorbidity and effort tolerance. Psychosomatics 31:197–203, 1990

Shumaker SA, Brownell A: Toward a theory of social support: closing conceptual gaps. Journal of Social Issues 40:11–36, 1984

Solomon SD, Smith EM, Robins LN, et al: Social involvement as a mediator of disaster-induced stress. Journal of Applied Social Psychology 17:1092–1112, 1987

Solomon SD, Regier DA, Burke JD: Role of perceived control in coping with disaster. Journal of Social Clinical Psychology 8:376–392, 1989

Solomon Z, Waysman M, Avitzur E, et al: Psychiatric symptomatology among wives of soldiers following combat stress reaction: the role of the social network and marital relations. Anxiety Research 4:213–223, 1991

Steinglass P, Gerrity E: Natural disasters and post-traumatic stress disorder: short-term versus long-term recovery in two disaster-affected communities. Journal of Applied Social Psychology 20:1746–1765, 1990

Stoller EP, Pugliesi KL: Other roles of caregivers: competing responsibilities or supportive resources. J Gerontol 44:231–238, 1989

Taylor SE: Health psychology: the science and the field. Am Psychol 45:40–50, 1990

Ursano RJ, McCaughey BG, Fullerton CS: The structure of human chaos, in Individual and Community Responses to Trauma and Disaster: The Structure of Human Chaos. Edited by Ursano RJ, McCaughey BG, Fullerton CS. London, Cambridge University Press, 1994, pp 403–410

Waigandt A, Wallace DL, Phelps L, et al: The impact of sexual assault on physical health status. J Trauma Stress 3:93–102, 1990

Wetzler HP, Ursano RJ: A positive association between physical health practices and psychological well-being. J Nerv Ment Dis 176: 280–283, 1988

Wilson JP, Raphael B (eds): International Handbook of Traumatic Stress Syndrome. New York, Plenum, 1993

Wingard D, Berkman LF: A multivariate analysis of health practices and social networks, in Social Support and Health. Edited by Cohen S, Syme SL. New York, Academic Press, 1985, pp 161–175

Chapter 5

Comorbidity of Posttraumatic Stress Disorder and Depression

Elie G. Karam, M.D.

The issue of causality in medicine is at the core of advances in the prevention and cure of disease. The public at large, in addition to researchers, closely monitors important advances (e.g., in molecular genetics and epidemiology), hoping that such advances will enable the medical profession to progressively conquer the ailments that plague humankind.

One "ailment" that goes beyond molecular understanding, yet seems to be linked with the human race, is war. This linkage is so strong that history books frequently boil down to the history of wars. We cannot predict whether wars will continue to ravage human societies, but each generation in almost every country has known war. Every war causes the destruction of property, the destruction of human lives, and extreme suffering.

My colleagues in the Clinical and Research Program, Department of Psychiatry, St. George Hospital, Beirut, Lebanon, and I have investigated war-related suffering since 1980. When we began our research, the Lebanon wars were in their sixth year; another 10 years passed before those wars ended. We were not alert to the diagnosis of posttraumatic stress disorder (PTSD), however, until we began to focus on war-related mental health literature (e.g., Curran 1988; Foy et al. 1984; Helzer et al. 1979; Keane et al. 1984; Loughrey et al. 1988; Mira 1939; Roussy and Lhermitte 1918; Yager et al. 1984).

Psychiatric and psychological researchers have identified some Axis I psychiatric syndromes that are comorbid with PTSD

I would like to thank Diantha B. Howard, Adel H. Chami, Jina C. Njeim, and Natalie A. Saikaly for their help in the analysis and preparation of this manuscript.

(Davidson and Fairbank 1992; Green et al. 1989; Karam et al. 1991; Keane and Wolfe 1990; Kulka et al. 1990, 1991; Maser and Cloninger 1990; Rundell et al. 1989; Ursano et al. 1995). In particular, mood disorders often coexist with PTSD. The literature is replete with studies of military personal (e.g., Green et al. 1990; Keane et al. 1991; Rosenheck et al. 1992; Solomon et al. 1990; Southwick et al. 1991) and clinical populations (e.g., Kinzie et al. 1990; Kroll et al. 1989); to our knowledge, however, no studies have assessed pre- and post-war civilian communities in a meticulous and prospective fashion.

In Beirut, our understanding of PTSD was influenced by what we saw in American movies—for instance, "flashbacks" or rampages of violence by soldiers just returned from Vietnam. Yet we did not see these symptoms in our patients, so we wondered whether these reactions were just dramatizations or simply did not exist in Lebanon. We rarely saw PTSD alone; when we did (e.g., in an emergency department or air raid shelter), we considered the symptoms to be "acute fear reactions," which usually disappeared with time. We regarded PTSD as a recollection of events that applied to a single trauma and thus would not apply to Lebanon, where people were repetitively traumatized by horrible wars that lasted for years.

Nevertheless, we have been alert to PTSD in our clinical practice for many years. In the Lebanon wars, which entailed chronic and enduring trauma, individuals experienced the feeling that the danger of a traumatic event and/or the sudden loss of a close loved one was inescapable. The wars led many people to feel that their loved ones were indeed vulnerable and that they had nowhere to run (e.g., in a massive "near miss" bomb experience).

Despite individual efforts over many years to discard the idea of mortality or helplessness, the overall experience of the Lebanon wars brought particular traumas roaring back to the consciousness of people who lived through the conflict, razing illusory walls that had helped them cope. Not only did they become scared; they also had no reason to expect the fear to stop. How could they know a traumatic event would not happen again? No words could dispel this frightening realization. Many of these people believed they escaped the trauma by mere chance and that it was only a matter of time before their turn came. With every shell that fell or every threat they heard, they found themselves alone. The arrows are falling all around us, but this time we are not in a show: those who are throwing the arrows want to hit us and not just draw nice circles around us.

People who lost a loved one thought—rightly so—that it could happen again and that next time, they themselves might not survive. What they thought would happen only to the unlucky or the elderly happened to everyone. Rules about how to avoid this dreaded fear fell one by one, day after day. Additional emotions emerged: Survivors became disenchanted with life and felt that their previous existence, when all was happy and secure, was meaningless. And the beads fall off one after the other.

The war trauma of Lebanon created a state of mind in which hope was diminished and the beauty of life was dampened by the horror of what happened and what may happen. In this situation, people often felt a tremendous rush of intrusive recollections, a decreased desire to participate in any active endeavor (including eating), and the pervasive feeling that they were alone.

These characteristics of trauma in Lebanon—coupled with the war's chronic, unrelenting, indiscriminate presence—highlight the importance of studying the comorbidity of PTSD with depression. In this chapter, I report the results of investigations by my colleagues and myself on the comorbidity of PTSD and depression in community samples in Lebanon.

STUDY METHODOLOGY

My colleagues and I began to examine the posttraumatic effects of the Lebanon war in 1989 (Phase I). We randomly selected a total of 658 individuals from four Lebanese communities differentially exposed to war (Karam 1992a). A team of psychologists trained in our center interviewed subjects in their homes using the Diagnostic Interview Schedule (DIS) (Robins et al. 1981) in its Arabic form (Karam et al. 1991) and the War Events Questionnaire (Karam 1992b).

In Phase I, we examined PTSD retrospectively over 13 years of war in a subgroup of subjects. Interviewing subjects about the consequences of 13 years of repeated trauma without retrospectively mixing responses to prior and subsequent traumatic events was difficult. Isolating specific traumatic episodes would have required a more clinical interview than the DIS, with a great deal of time devoted to comparing pre- and posttrauma.

We tried meticulously to stay alert to the potential inaccuracies and distortions of retrospective recall (Norris and Kaniasty 1992). We believed that unless PTSD was massive and caused substantial dysfunction, recalling specific events while living in a chronic war zone would be difficult. A civilian who was exposed to a mortar shell explosion would, expectedly, keep thinking about it for several days—"expectedly" because besides the specific episode, shells were falling before and kept falling afterwards. Yet, we also would expect such an individual to have an exaggerated startle reflex, be hypervigilant, and avoid situations and places that reminded him or her of the trauma. Following the natural inclination to avoid dangerously exposed areas, for example, the people of Lebanon learned new behaviors: not to stay in top floors, not to come home or wander the streets after dark, to avoid specific areas in and around Beirut, to stay away from windows, to check on the news before moving around, and to rapidly cross specific streets.

We completed the Phase I subject interviews a week or two before the eruption of the Aoun-Geagea War—the most ferocious chapter of the Lebanon wars. Hardest hit were two communities that had been part of our Phase I interviews. With the help of a rapid grant from the National Institute of Mental Health, we initiated Phase II of our Lebanon war studies.

In Phase II (conducted in 1991), we reinterviewed 234 subjects within 6 months of the end of the Aoun-Geagea conflict, the last of the Lebanon wars (peace has settled in Lebanon since October 1990). Subjects on whom we had previous lifetime data were reinterviewed by the same interviewers that had seen them 14–17 months earlier. We assessed subjects for 1-year depression and 1-year PTSD using the same interview measures as in Phase I (DIS and War Events Questionnaire) but focused on the period after February 1990—that is, after the conclusion of Phase I.

Our PTSD interview consisted of the following approach: We first checked on all war events the subject might have been exposed to in the past year; we then reviewed each event, assessing the subject for PTSD symptoms that followed or were exacerbated by that event. We inquired about the beginning and the end of each symptom. We started each interview with the event that the subject rated worst and continued event by event until the subject had less than the minimal PTSD symptom for at least two consecutive events.

RESULTS

Depression

For this study, my colleagues and I used DSM-III-R (American Psychiatric Association 1987). The DSM-III-R definition of major depression excluded bereavement-related episodes unless they are very severe or last more than 1 year. A community study (Karam 1994) suggested that exclusion of bereavement-related depressions from major depression (if they satisfy at least the minimal criteria) may not be well founded. For consistency, we classified depressions as *major depression* (MD) if they satisfied the DSM-III-R criteria; *any precipitant major depression* (AMD) included depressive episodes that met the criteria for major depression regardless of their precipitant. *Bereavement depressions* (BD) were episodes related to bereavement that satisfied other DSM-III-R criteria.

Table 5–1 shows the prevalence of depression in our subjects. Our data suggest an important relationship between war exposure and depression. The subjects' place of residence per se was not as important as the level of exposure to actual war events (E. Karam, unpublished manuscript, August 1995). There were no significant

Table 5–1. Lifetime and 1-year prevalence of depression and PTSD

	Lifetime MD	Lifetime AMD	1-Year MD	1-Year AMD	1-Year BD[a]	1-Year PTSD
Males	30.3	34.3	32.3	38.4	6.1	9.1
Females	28.9	34.1	34.1	46.7	12.6	11.1
Total	29.5	34.2	33.3	43.2	9.8	10.3

Note. Values given are percentages. MD = major depression; AMD = any precipitant major depression; BD = bereavement depression; PTSD = posttraumatic stress disorder.
[a]Pure bereavement depression.

differences between males and females, even for the bloodiest year of the wars. The 1-year prevalence of depression (MD and AMD) was nearly the same as the lifetime prevalence of depression.

Posttraumatic Stress Disorder

Table 5–1 also shows the 1-year prevalence of PTSD. Again, there were no substantial differences between males and females; 10.3% of all subjects had experienced PTSD since the onset of the last chapter of the war.

Exposure to War and Comorbidity

Our findings indicate a robust relationship between exposure to war in Phase II and the development of comorbidity (see Figure 5–1). The relationship between Phase II war exposure and comorbidity approaches significance ($P = 0.089$) for the DSM-III-R definition of MD but is quite significant ($P = 0.0074$) for AMD. The more the subjects were exposed to war, the more they simultaneously developed PTSD and depression.

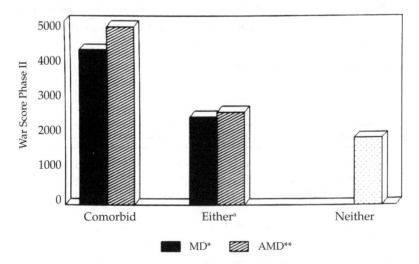

Figure 5–1. Comorbidity of posttraumatic stress disorder and depression: exposure in Phase II. MD = major depression; AMD = any precipitant major depression.
[a]Either depression or PTSD alone; *$P = .0899$; **$P = .0074$.

Prior Exposure to War and Comorbidity on Reexposure

Does war sensitize individuals to further exposure? Does it protect them? To determine whether there was any difference in prior war exposure (Phase I) between those who developed both syndromes (depression and PTSD) and those who developed either or neither on reexposure (Phase II), we considered both definitions of depression (Figure 5–2). Prior exposure (Phase I) seemed not only to predispose individuals to individual syndromes (i.e., MD or PTSD) on reexposure (P = 0.079; one-way analysis of variance), but also appeared to increase the likelihood of a comorbid state (i.e., MD and PTSD). This relationship did not obtain for AMD, however.

Depression and PTSD in Phase II

The prevalence of PTSD increased with the presence of depression (Figure 5–3); this correlation is significant for AMD. Levels of significance (versus not depressed) were P = 0.10 for MD, P = 0.0019 for AMD, and P = 0.0000 for BD.

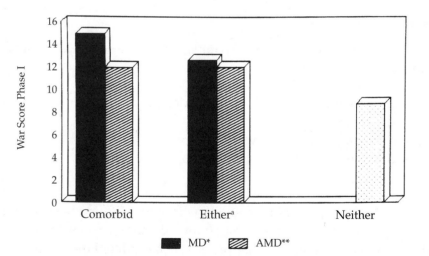

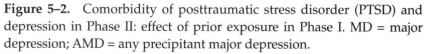

Figure 5–2. Comorbidity of posttraumatic stress disorder (PTSD) and depression in Phase II: effect of prior exposure in Phase I. MD = major depression; AMD = any precipitant major depression.
[a] Either depression or PTSD alone. *One-way analysis of variance P = .0795.
**One-way analysis of variance P = .1641.

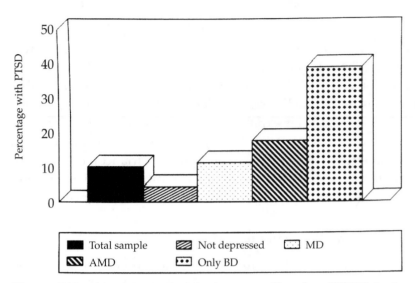

Figure 5–3. 1-year posttraumatic stress disorder (PTSD) in 1-year depression subjects. MD = major depression; AMD = any precipitant major depression; BD = bereavement depression.

Nature of War Events

The war events we considered in our study can be subdivided into three groups:

1. Damage to property of interviewee or a person very close to the interviewee
2. Physical injuries to self/very close person
3. Kidnapping of self/very close person.

We also regarded witnessing these events as a factor.

Except for physical injuries to self, war scores differed regarding whether the subject simply knew about the war event, saw it from afar, or was present when it happened. We considered the category of war events that gave rise to PTSD: More than half (58.3%) of the subjects who had PTSD exhibited symptoms after fatal war events, 20.3% of fatal events were followed by PTSD, and 21.2% of subjects who had experienced fatal events had PTSD. For reference, 28.2% of the subjects reported a fatal event in the past year (Phase II).

As Tables 5–2 and 5–3 show, the nature of the event seemed to have a major correlation to the comorbidity of PTSD and depression; this correlation, however, might simply reflect the sharp increase in PTSD following fatal events. The correlation appears for both definitions of depression: 85% of subjects who had PTSD secondary to a fatal event had depression (AMD), but the percentage was still high (64%) even when we restricted our definition of depression to MD. Nevertheless, half of the comorbidity cases were lost when we used MD rather than AMD.

Previous Depression

Because our study also was prospective, we examined the relationship between depression (in Phase I) before the bloodiest chapter of the Lebanon wars and the likelihood of comorbid PTSD and depression in the follow-up period (Phase II), after heavy exposure

Table 5–2.   Nature of events: 1-year PTSD and 1-year MD

	No MD, no PTSD	MD	MD alone	PTSD	PTSD alone	Comorbid
Without	63.7	32.7	30.4	6.0	3.6	2.4
With	51.5	34.8	27.3	21.2	13.6	7.6

Note.   Values given are percentages. MD = major depression; PTSD = posttraumatic stress disorder; without = subjects without fatal events, N = 168; with = subjects with fatal events, N = 66.

Table 5–3.   Nature of events: 1-year PTSD and 1-year AMD

	No AMD, no PTSD	AMD	AMD alone	PTSD	PTSD alone	Comorbid
Without	56.5	41.1	37.5	6.0	2.4	3.6
With	48.5	48.5	30.3	21.2	3.0	18.2

Note.   Values given are percentages. AMD = any precipitant major depression; PTSD = posttraumatic stress disorder; without = subjects without fatal events, N = 168; with = subjects with fatal events, N = 66.

(Table 5–4). The correlation between depression in Phase I and depression, PTSD, or comorbidity in Phase II was significant ($P = 0.000$) for both MD and AMD.

These data confirm previous findings (Karam 1994) that MD and AMD have equal predictive power for subsequent development of depression (any type). Notably, the prevalence of PTSD, MD, or AMD doubled in Phase II when depression was present in Phase I; comorbidity (MD + PTSD, AMD + PTSD) increased three- to fivefold (see Table 5–4). These results could be because of simple arithmetic: If the probability of PTSD and depression increases for subjects with previous depression, then naturally the probability of a comorbid state also would increase.

However, this finding also might mean that PTSD is related to depression more than psychiatrists previously thought. According to our current findings, there is a relationship between mood disorders and PTSD in war. Research exploring possible precipitants of depression might shed further light on this point. The issue is important because the definition of trauma remains hazy—although it has become more precise in DSM-IV (American Psychiatric Association 1994).

Final Predictors of Depression and PTSD

A previous study (E. Karam, unpublished manuscript, August 1995) found that depression was related to exposure to war. We thought

Table 5–4. Previous depression (Phase I) and comorbidity on reexposure (Phase II)

			Phase II		
			MD &		AMD &
Phase I	PTSD	MD	PTSD	AMD	PTSD
No previous depression	7.1	27.1	2.1	31.8	4.5
Previous MD	17.4	55.9	10.2	62.3	14.5
Previous AMD	16.3	58.2	9.0	65.0	13.8

Note. Values are given as percentages. MD = major depression; AMD = any precipitant major depression; PTSD = posttraumatic stress disorder.

that prior depression (Phase I) might predict depression and PTSD (Phase II) only through a common variable such as higher exposure in Phase I, which itself could predict more exposure in Phase II. Therefore, we introduced in a logistic regression the following variables: exposure in Phase I, depression (MD, AMD) in Phase I, exposure in Phase II, fatal events in Phase II, and depression in Phase I x fatal events in Phase II. Table 5–5 shows that the risk of developing a comorbid state increased six- to eightfold if a subject had previous depression (Phase I) and experienced a fatal war event (Phase II).

Summary

Our results point to the rise of two major syndromes after war: PTSD and depression. Previous symptomatology (i.e., prior depression) and direct intense exposure to war (i.e., experiencing a fatal event) were the most important predictors; because of the small sample size, the negative predictive ability is more apparent than the positive one. This finding echoes similar prospective studies by Smith et al. (1986) and Robins et al. (1986) on another type of disaster (flood).

War alone did not stand as an independent factor in our analyses. The interaction between previous psychiatric comorbidity (Phase I) and exposure to war (fatal events) in Phase II was significant, however.

CONCLUSION

Trauma and PTSD raise issues similar to those regarding bereavement and depression (noted earlier). With regard to PTSD, we

---

Table 5–5. Predictors of PTSD and depression comorbidity: logistic regression

Variable	Standard beta	Standard error	Significance (P)	Odds ratio
MD x fatal Phase II*	1.7917	0.7564	.0179	5.9996
AMD x fatal Phase II**	2.0737	0.5887	.0004	7.9541

Note. PTSD = posttraumatic stress disorder; MD = major depression; AMD = any precipitant major depression
*loglikelihood = –36.88; P = .0331. **loglikelihood = –58.51; P = .0012.

grapple with the definition of a precipitant; with regard to depression, we wonder whether we have the right to omit some specific precipitant. The results of our study suggest that PTSD and depression coexist often under extreme circumstances. This finding highlights issues of precipitators and separate entities in psychiatric nosology: Does comorbidity increase only because PTSD increases in itself, or are we dealing with one "entity" precipitated by a traumatic event—a specific entity that combines elements of depression and PTSD?

REFERENCES

American Psychiatric Association: Diagnostic and Statistical Manual of Mental Disorders, 3rd Edition, Revised. Washington, DC, American Psychiatric Association, 1987

American Psychiatric Association: Diagnostic and Statistical Manual of Mental Disorders, 4th Edition. Washington, DC, American Psychiatric Association, 1994

Curran PS: Psychiatric aspects of terrorist violence: Northern Ireland 1969–1987. Br J Psychiatry 153:470–475, 1988

Davidson JRT, Fairbank JA: The epidemiology of posttraumatic stress disorder, in Posttraumatic Stress Disorder: DSM-IV and Beyond. Edited by Davidson JRT, Foa EB. Washington, DC, American Psychiatric Press, 1992, pp 147–169

Foy DW, Rueger DB, Sipprelle RC, et al: Etiology of posttraumatic stress disorder in Vietnam veterans: analysis of premilitary, military and combat exposure influences. J Consult Clin Psychiatry 52:79–87, 1984

Green BL, Lindy JD, Grace MC, et al: Multiple diagnosis in posttraumatic stress disorder: the role of war stressors. J Nerv Ment Dis 177: 329–335, 1989

Green BL, Grace MC, Lindy JD, et al: War stressor and symptom persistence in posttraumatic stress disorder. Journal of Anxiety Disorders 4:31–39, 1990

Helzer JE, Robins LN, Wish ED: Depression in Vietnam veterans and Sicilian controls. Am J Psychiatry 136:526–529, 1979

Karam EG: Depression et Guerres du Liban: Methodologie, d'une Recherche. Revue Annales St. Joseph University (Beirut) 131:99–106, 1992a

Karam EG: The War Events Questionnaire. New York, United Nations, April 1992b

Karam EG: The nosological status of bereavement-related depressions. Br J Psychiatry 165:524–529, 1994

Karam EG, Barakeh M, Karam AN, et al: The Arabic DIS. Revue Medicale Libanaise 3, 1991

Keane TM, Wolfe J: Comorbidity in post-traumatic stress disorder: an analysis of community and clinical studies. Journal of Applied Social Psychology 20:1776–1788, 1990

Keane TM, Malloy PF, Fairbank JA: Empirical development of an MMPI subscale for the assessment of combat-related PTSD. J Consult Clin Psychol 52:888–891, 1984

Keane TM, Litz BT, Weathers F, et al: New methods for assessing PTSD: research and clinical approaches. Paper presented at The Reality of Trauma in Everyday Life: Implications for Intervention and Policy. Seventh annual convention of the International Society for Traumatic Stress Studies, Washington, DC, October 1991

Kinzie JD, Boehenliem JK, Leung PK, et al: The prevalence of posttraumatic stress disorder and its clinical significance among Southeast Asian refugees. Am J Psychiatry 147:913–917, 1990

Kroll J, Habenicht M, Mackenzie T, et al: Depression and posttraumatic stress disorder in Southeast Asian refugees. Am J Psychiatry 146:12, 1989

Kulka RA, Schlenger WE, Fairbank JA, et al: Trauma and the Vietnam War Generation. New York, Brunner/Mazel, 1990

Kulka RA, Schlenger WE, Fairbank JA, et al: Assessment of posttraumatic stress disorder in the community: prospects and pitfalls from recent studies of Vietnam veterans. Psychological Assessment: A Journal of Consulting and Clinical Psychology 3:547–560, 1991

Loughrey GC, Bell P, Roodyand RJ, et al: Post-traumatic stress disorder and civil violence in Northern Ireland. Br J Psychiatry 153:554–560, 1988

Maser JD, Cloninger CR: Comorbidity of Mood and Psychiatric Disorders. Washington, DC, American Psychiatric Press, 1990

Mira E: Psychiatric disturbances during the Spanish Civil War. BMJ 281:975, 1939

Norris F, Kaniasty K: Reliability of delayed self-reports in disaster research. J Trauma Stress 5:575–588, 1992

Robins LN, Helzer JE, Croughan J, et al: National Institute of Mental Health Diagnostic Interview Schedule: its history, characteristics, and validity. Arch Gen Psychiatry 38:381–389, 1981

Robins LN, Fishbach RL, Smith EM, et al: Impact of disaster on previously assessed mental health, in Disaster Stress Studies: New Methods and Findings. Edited by Shore JE. Washington, DC, American Psychiatric Press, 1986, pp 22–48

Rosenheck R, Becnel H, Blank AS, et al: Returning Persian Gulf Troops: First-year findings. Report of the Department of Veterans Affairs to the United States Congress on the psychological effects of the Persian Gulf War, 1992

Roussy G, Lhermitte J: The Psychoneuroses of War. Edited by Turner WA. London, University of London Press, 1918

Rundell JR, Ursano RJ, Holloway HC, et al: Psychiatric responses to trauma. Hosp Comm Psychiatry 40:68–74, 1989

Smith EM, Robins LN, Przybeck TR, et al: Psychosocial consequences of a disaster, in Disaster Stress Studies: New Methods and Findings. Edited by Shore JE. Washington, DC, American Psychiatric Press, 1986, pp 50–76

Solomon Z, Bleich A, Koslowsky M, et al: Post-traumatic stress disorder: issues of co-morbidity. J Psychiatr Res 25:110–117, 1990

Southwick SM, Yehuda R, Giller EL, Jr: Characterization of depression in war related post-traumatic stress disorder. Am J Psychiatry 148:179–183, 1991

Ursano RJ, Fullerton CS, Bhartiya V, et al: Longitudinal assessment of posttraumatic stress disorder and depression after exposure to traumatic death. J Nerv Ment Dis 183:36–43, 1995

Yager T, Laufer R, Gallops M: Some problems associated with war experience in men of the Vietnam generation. Arch Gen Psychiatry 41:327–333, 1984

Chapter 6

War-Related Psychopathology in Kuwait: An Assessment of War-Related Mental Health Problems

Lars Weisæth, M.D., Ph.D.

W ar is a complex mixture of psychologically traumatic events. Standard psychiatric textbooks (e.g., Kaplan et al. 1980) limit their coverage of war psychiatry to syndromes related to combat or prisoner-of-war (POW) experiences. Recent studies however, have expanded this scope considerably (Ursano and Norwood 1996).

People in different countries view war differently, depending on their national history. Some Western nations (e.g., the United States and Canada) have regarded war primarily as a cluster of events affecting military personnel on foreign soil—by no means forgetting, however, the grief suffered by POWs' next of kin and families of fallen soldiers. Citizens of other countries (e.g., Great Britain and Australia) have experienced additional war-related traumas, such as having homes destroyed by enemy bombs. Still other nations have endured surprise invasion followed by partial occupation (France); full occupation of the entire country, with the legal government in exile (Norway); or full occupation of the country, with the government captive (Denmark). Finally, neutral countries (e.g., Sweden and Switzerland) have escaped first-hand experience of war altogether, although they have lived through periods of internal strife, insecurity, reduced living standards because of food and fuel rationing, and steady pressure to admit and assist refugees from occupied countries. Each of these kinds of experiences leaves a trail of traumatic effects.

Experiences suffered by the people of Kuwait during the Persian Gulf War of 1990–1991 illustrate a wide variety of war traumas. This tiny oil nation thus constitutes a virtual laboratory for studies of postwar psychopathology. Kuwait's war experiences offer material for a wider analytical conception of war trauma that draws on a time-phase model.

Nations that suffer sudden invasion leading to total occupation—as Kuwait endured in 1990–1991—experience most aspects of war trauma: threat, attack, invasion, occupation, liberation, postwar legal actions against collaborators and war criminals, and finally peace, with the reestablishment of national institutions. Whether preannounced or unexpected, armed invasions tend to cause a variety of distinct psychiatric casualties (Eitinger 1990); occupation following military defeat is a multifaceted, complex trauma for the national population. Different groups of people will be exposed to unique stressors; psychiatrists have not thoroughly studied most of these stressors with regard to their mental health consequences. Liberation may entail reversal of some previously defined roles: although most people would not consider traitors to be victims, for example, they may suffer severe psychopathological consequences as an effect of having been on the "wrong" side.

WAR AND MENTAL HEALTH— A COMPLEX RELATIONSHIP

The relationship between war and mental health is complex. Not all war experiences lead to problems; some may even have positive effects. During the Nazi occupation of Norway, for example, the prevalence of certain types of psychoses decreased 15% (Ødegård 1954). Mental health problems may be more common in threatened areas than in actual combat zones, where people cannot afford the luxury of fear (Punamaki 1990). However, in the only study to date of an ongoing occupation, my colleagues and I found high degrees of distress within Palestinian society in Gaza, the West Bank, and Arab Jerusalem, despite the relatively moderate nature of Israel's occupation (Giacaman et al. 1993).

Because of the psychological complexity of war and the fact that the line between military and civilian exposures during an occupation is less distinct, psychiatrists must be alert to many potentially affected groups within the general population. For example, segments of an occupied nation's population may spend extended periods of time in exile: war often entails mass migration of refugees into and out of the country, as well as internal refugees (often called displaced persons). Military forces undergoing training on foreign soil and border runners—including sea and land pilots—who keep clandestine traffic going between occupied territories and the outside world also present special concerns. Psychiatrists must not overlook these high-risk groups.

After World War II, for example, merchant seamen (Norway alone had 40,000) often were neglected. These sailors wore no military uniforms, and they were not considered "real" war participants. Yet they made crucial contributions to the allied war effort by transporting arms, ammunition, fuel, provisions, and troops to the battlefields; many were exposed to greater traumatic stress than individuals in uniform. These seamen were exposed to severe uncertainty for 5 years, waiting for the torpedo they hoped would never come. These wartime experiences led to severe mental health consequences (Askevold 1976/1977).

VARYING SEVERITY OF OCCUPATION

An occupying power may treat the suppressed population in various ways; occupations vary in severity along a continuum. At one end of the spectrum, the occupier may try to enlist the local population in support of its efforts—possibly based on ideological, ethnic, religious, or other criteria. In such cases, the pressure of an occupation may be rather moderate, with severe retaliation reserved for overt resistance only. The other end of the spectrum can include a completely enslaved population, genocide, and the total extermination of large subcultures; this pattern is familiar from the history of totalitarian regimes, as well as recent wars such as those in Bosnia and Rwanda.

Stressful events—traumatic exposures with resulting psychopathological effects—abound all along this continuum. These stressors include loss of freedom, suspension of law, threats to national or ethnic identity, disruption of national institutions, political oppression, terror, abductions, hostage-taking, murder, summary execution, rape, torture, arbitrary arrests and imprisonment, disappearances, splitting up of families, and loss of close relatives. Various forms of active and passive resistance—"illegal" or clandestine news services, civil disobedience, life-in-hiding, infiltration, secret agents, double agents, sabotage, intelligence services, and a variety of armed elements and secret military forces—also may entail stressful events and effects.

KUWAIT: LAND AND PEOPLE

Kuwait covers an area of about 17,800 square kilometers (about 11,000 square miles); the country extends approximately 200 km north to south and 170 km east to west. In 1990 Kuwait had a total population of about 2 million people; its population is almost entirely urban (94%). At the time of the invasion, Kuwaitis enjoyed universal schooling and a high literacy rate (82%). The birth rate was relatively high and the death rate low; infant mortality rate was 14 per 1,000 (World Health Organization 1992).

The composition of the Kuwaiti population is an important consideration in any analysis of the nation's war-related psychopathology. Before the invasion, Kuwaiti citizens—that is, individuals of Kuwaiti origin—constituted about 40% of the total population (World Health Organization 1992). Obtaining Kuwaiti citizenship is extremely difficult for foreigners; nevertheless, as of 1985, 38% of the population originated in other Arab countries—of whom at least half were Palestinians—and 21% in Asia. The Arab, non-Kuwaiti population included more than 100,000 Bedouins with a long history of residency on Kuwaiti territory; because of their seasonal migrations across national borders, they are not recognized as citizens of any state. The non-Kuwaiti population consisted largely of guest workers who had settled in the country in recent decades. Some of these inhabitants fled during the war and occupation. Many of these noncitizens have not been allowed to return since the liberation; others have been encouraged or forced to leave.

PHASES OF WAR

The characteristics of any war are defined by its timing, particular war events, specific traumas of each phase, and psychological effects. The phases of war include peace prior to war, threat, attack, invasion, occupation, liberation, postwar activities, and postwar peace. The war in Kuwait followed this pattern (Keesing's Record of World Events 1990, 1991).

Prewar Peace

Kuwait has been a sovereign state since 1921. For many years—living off its vast oil resources—it had the world's highest GNP per capita. Before the Iraqi invasion, Kuwait enjoyed peace with its neighbors and pursued a peaceful foreign policy.

Threat

Impoverished by its long war with Iran (1980–1988), Iraq launched strong verbal attacks on Kuwait and other Persian Gulf states in 1989–1990, claiming that Kuwait had "stolen" oil worth $2.4 billion and threatening to retrieve the value of the stolen oil. Iraq deployed 30,000 elite troops on the Kuwaiti border, with more troops from its army of 1 million men close behind.

Yet most Kuwaitis did not believe that Iraq's threats were serious, particularly because political negotiations were being held in Jiddah, Saudi Arabia. On August 1, 1990, however, the negotiations broke down, with no solution in sight.

Attack

The Iraqi surprise attack on Kuwait took place in the early morning hours of August 2, 1990. Kuwaiti border guards were overrun by Iraqi troops, who claimed that they had been invited by Kuwaiti revolutionaries.

Invasion

Within 8 hours of the initial attack, Iraqi troops had taken all important positions and were in full control of the country. The Iraqi invaders suspended Kuwait's legal institutions and drove its head of state into exile. In response, the United Nations Security Council adopted Resolution 660 calling for an immediate and unconditional Iraqi withdrawal. Further resolutions laid the foundation for the allied ultimatum and subsequent Operation Desert Storm to liberate Kuwait.

Occupation

The Iraqi occupation of Kuwait lasted from August 2, 1990, to February 26, 1991. On August 25, 1990, approximately 100,000 Iraqi soldiers were in Kuwait; Iraq proclaimed Kuwait the 19th Iraqi governorate on August 28, 1990. During the occupation, Iraq held several thousand Western citizens hostage, under varying degrees of hardship.

Following the invasion, the international community imposed sanctions on Iraq. After the United Nations ultimatum, allied troops gathered in Saudi Arabia in preparation for Operation Desert Storm. Uniting under mandates from the United Nations Security Council, these allied forces had four "just causes" for evicting Iraq from Kuwait:

- Kuwait was a small nation under an unprovoked attack by a powerful and militant neighboring state.
- The allied forces intended to stop a well-known aggressor in the area. (Iraq's long war with Iran contributed to this attitude.)
- The international community wanted to prevent nuclear, biological, and chemical warfare and the proliferation of such weapons. (United Nations investigation teams later confirmed the danger.)
- The allies aimed to protect the principle of free trade of oil.

The allied counterattack on Iraq formally began on January 16, 1991, with heavy bombing of Baghdad and other centers. The Desert Storm land offensive against Iraq was launched on February 24, 1991. Iraqi forces fled Kuwait City on February 25, taking with them about 5,000 Kuwaiti citizens as hostages, and on February 26, the Kuwaiti resistance movement claimed to be in control of the capital. Iraqi leader Saddam Hussein announced Iraqi "victory" and the start of Iraqi troop withdrawal from Kuwait; on the same day, the emir of Kuwait placed the country under martial law for a period of 3 months.

Liberation

On February 27, 1991, Saudi Arabian troops entered Kuwait City. Although the Kuwaiti army's 6th brigade originally had been chosen to spearhead the troops liberating the city, fear that returning Kuwaiti soldiers might seek revenge on the capital's 240,000 Palestinian inhabitants for atrocities committed by Iraqi forces during the occupation led the allied forces to reconsider. Before the allies arrived, all of Kuwait's 950 producing oil wells were set ablaze or damaged by Iraqi sabotage, causing catastrophic water and air pollution.

More than 7,000 Kuwaitis had died during the occupation; an estimated 17,000 were held captive and subjected to torture in camps in Iraq and Kuwait.

Allied military operations were suspended on February 28, 1991, and a formal cease-fire was signed on March 3. The war and occupation had lasted 208 days (approximately 7 months).

Postwar Period

The immediate postwar period was characterized by the return of Kuwaitis who had served in the free forces or had been refugees in exile during the occupation. Black smoke from hundreds of burning oil wells covered the sky and caused breathing problems. Most public institutions had been disrupted. Only a few hospitals were operating, with severe shortages of equipment, personnel, and water. Many buildings were in ruins. Thousands of people were seriously affected by their grueling experiences during the war and occupation. Many were mourning their dead and searching for missing relatives.

Postwar Peace

Kuwait was still struggling to return to a fully normal peace situation 3 years after the successful termination of the occupation. Among the factors causing delays in the return to normalcy were the profusion of deadly mines left behind, ongoing political conflicts, and the continued threat from Iraq. These problems illustrate the severe and prolonged difficulties in overcoming the effects of even a relatively brief war. However, the military liberation of Kuwait has had some positive effects on Middle East geopolitics: Kuwait's advance toward political emancipation may be the region's most immediate and important test case for democratization (Green 1993).

WORLD HEALTH ORGANIZATION MISSION

In December 1990, the Kuwaiti government in exile asked the World Health Organization (WHO) to come into Kuwait as soon as possible after liberation to assess the health situation and advise the government regarding health services and human rights. Immediately following the liberation in February 1991, the United Nations dispatched two missions to Kuwait: a "humanitarian" mission and a "health and health hazards" mission. The health mission identified 10 major health problems, including posttraumatic stress disorder (PTSD) and other psychological problems related to the trauma of war and occupation.

An emergency health plan was developed for the first 3 months, and WHO assigned a liaison officer in Kuwait as a personal representative of the Director General to assist in the implementation of the plan. The liaison officer worked with the Division of Mental Health at WHO Headquarters in Geneva and WHO's East Mediterranean Regional Office to establish a consultant mission to advise the Kuwaiti government regarding the mental health consequences of the war.

A five-member WHO team—comprising three Norwegian psychiatrists with special expertise in the problems of war and disaster, including a woman with expertise in problems associated with sexual violence; an Egyptian psychiatrist with special expertise in Arab and Islamic culture, as well as national mental health planning; and a WHO staff member[1]—spent 2 weeks in Kuwait in October 1991. This mission had several goals:

- To examine the nature and extent of war-related mental health problems in Kuwait following its occupation
- To make recommendations on how health services and other social sectors could be strengthened to respond to such problems
- To suggest specific activities in response to these problems

---

[1]The WHO team consisted of Lars Weisæth, M.D. (leader); Solveig Dahl, M.D.; Paal Herlofsen, M.D.; Muhammed Shalaan, M.D.; and John Orley, Senior Medical Officer, Division of Mental Health, World Health Organization.

The WHO team recommended an epidemiological survey to identify groups suffering from postwar psychopathology (WHO 1992). This survey would serve as the basis for systematic preventive and therapeutic interventions.

NATIONAL EPIDEMIOLOGICAL STUDY

The epidemiological study took place in June 1993—almost 2 $1/2$ years after liberation (Al-Hammadi et al. 1993). The investigators made contact with several Kuwaiti ministries (e.g., Public Health), the National Association for Defense of War Victims, nongovernmental institutions, and expert personnel. They interviewed key informants and individuals directly affected by the war including families with missing members, prisoners of war, torture survivors, patients and personnel from local primary care and mental health services clinics, teachers, student leaders, social workers, nurses, neurologists, surgeons, plastic surgeons, ophthalmologists, and 6th-year medical students in their psychiatric term. Many interviewees shared personal and professional war-related experiences.

From a mental health standpoint, when the war ended the situation in Kuwait satisfied the definition of a disaster. The needs overwhelmed the resources; only 10% of Kuwait's prewar medical personnel remained in the country.

No nation, after an occupation, has provided satisfactory health services for the entire population. This pattern primarily reflects a lack of scientific knowledge and resources, as well as denial and avoidance of problems. The relative magnitude of Kuwait's war experience, the small size of the country and its population, and the extent and quality of prewar health services—coupled with a steady increase in knowledge about the treatment and prevention of traumatic stress responses—suggested, however, that Kuwait might be in a position to provide such services. The main limiting factor probably was the shortage of qualified mental health professionals. The epidemiological study documented that only a small percentage of Kuwaitis with a diagnosis of PTSD had been offered treatment (Al-Hammadi et al. 1993).

The duration of exposure to war stress among Kuwaiti citizens offered an important predictor and a basis for scaling the exposure.

The 208-day duration of the occupation—approximately 7 months—implies important risks to long-term health. Follow-up studies of war victims exposed to extreme stress have shown that continuous exposure of more than 6 months, particularly when such stress is uncontrollable and unpredictable, not only leads to increased general and psychiatric morbidity that can last for decades but also may be accompanied by increased mortality; many of these health problems appear after a period of latency (Eitinger and Strøm 1973).

Kuwaitis who were severely exposed during the occupation were at risk for long-term health problems that would be difficult or impossible to identify soon after the war. Nevertheless, risk groups could be established on the basis of the type and duration of exposure. The population comprised three exposure groups: those who stayed in Kuwait during the entire 7-month occupation, those who escaped at some point during the occupation, and those who were abroad at the time of the invasion and did not experience the occupation directly.

Psychiatrists often assess the mental health effects of psychic trauma according to presumed cause (see Table 6–1). Combinations of causes may complicate the analysis of likely effects. Although researchers have not thoroughly studied the health effects of the various causes, observations support this classification—human malice, for example, causes more severe effects than the other factors listed in Table 6–1 (Weisæth 1989). The deliberate murder of a family member, for example, would cause more psychopathology than deaths caused by negligence, such as lack of medical care.

Intentionality provides one explanation for inconsistency in reports of Kuwaiti war casualties. Direct Iraqi aggression caused the deaths of 1,500 Kuwaitis (0.23% of a population of 650,000 Kuwaitis); Kuwaiti documents referred to these victims as "martyrs." The higher estimate of 7,000 deaths may represent the total number of war-related deaths (including deaths from other causes during the period of the occupation).

Findings: Trauma and Psychological Effects

The primary rationale for a time-phase model is its predictive validity concerning the risk for immediate, subacute, and long-term

Table 6–1. Mental health effects of psychic trauma

Presumed cause	Likely effects
Natural cause	Accepted as accidental deaths, fatalistic acceptance, etc.
Technological failure	Blame for loss of control, preventive measures, etc.
Human negligence	Blame and loss of credibility, etc.
Human malice	Fight (aggression), flight (fear), surrender (shame), humiliation, narcissistic injuries, hatred, eventually revenge, cycles of violence

posttraumatic psychopathology. This model is particularly useful in assessing PTSD.

Prewar Peace

Until 1990 Kuwait's national policy had been to prevent and avoid war. Despite strong verbal threats from Baghdad during July 1990, Kuwaitis did not believe an attack might be imminent. A general state of unpreparedness among the military and the civilian population characterized the country's psychological status before the war.

Threat

The threat phase was characterized by a classic lack of understanding regarding the seriousness of Saddam Hussein's threats. Despite copious information on troop movements and other activities, Kuwaitis evinced a general disbelief in the imminent danger of war. This false sense of security derived not from a lack of information but from a failure in interpretation; Kuwaitis displayed insufficient arousal and vigilance. This type of denial is a well-known vulnerability factor, increasing the risk of severe shock and subsequent PTSD.

Attack

Few Kuwaitis experienced the Iraqi attack personally, and few lives were lost. Most Kuwaitis woke up during the night or in the morning to the sights and sounds of war: gunfire, tanks, and an overwhelming number of hostile foreign troops. As an indication of the population's sustained denial and wishful thinking, many reported that they initially believed that the troops were Kuwaiti forces on maneuvers.

Invasion

The Iraqi invasion began at 2 a.m. on August 2, 1990; 8 hours later, the invaders closed the borders. The country had been overrun and was largely outside Kuwaiti control. Thus, the invasion itself was of short duration. Lacking previous war experience, the population was caught unprepared and trapped suddenly. The presence of a large, unexpected invading army came as a complete shock to Kuwaitis; many experienced the invasion as an inescapable shock trauma, a well-known risk factor for the development of PTSD.

At the time of the invasion, the Kuwaiti segment of the population was reduced from 650,000 to approximately 400,000–450,000 because many Kuwaiti citizens were on vacations abroad; many non-Kuwaiti residents also were visiting abroad. Yet 89% of the subjects in the epidemiological sample reported that they were in Kuwait on August 2, 1990 (Al-Hammadi et al. 1993).

Because the invasion happened at night, family members who stayed in Kuwait generally remained together and did not split up. Nevertheless, a considerable number of family members were separated from next of kin at the time of the invasion. As a result, separation problems were an important element of the psychological situation from the beginning of the war.

Most of the modest number of casualties during the invasion involved military personnel. Although the indiscriminate use of military power and violence exposed all individuals to some risk, the Kuwaiti portion of the population was at greater risk than other nationalities. Some Kuwaitis managed to escape at this early stage. Brief reactive psychoses developed during this phase of the war; such disorders commonly result from surprise invasions (Eitinger 1990). In sum, Kuwait's psychological state was characterized by disbelief, widespread confusion, paralysis, and panic-stricken flight, as well as some psychotic reactions.

Occupation

Before the invasion, Kuwait and Iraq had enjoyed close ties. During the Iran-Iraq war, the Kuwaiti government had supported Iraq financially. Intermarriage between Kuwaiti and Iraqi families was common. Kuwaitis therefore felt a deep sense of betrayal when these former allies and kin suddenly turned against them.

In the initial stages of the occupation, non-Kuwaiti segments of the population—particularly people who came from nations and political movements supporting Iraq in the war (especially Palestinians)—distanced themselves from Kuwaiti citizens. Kuwaitis found that two populations—Iraqi and Palestinian—that they had previously regarded as friends had turned aggressively against them. For many Kuwaitis, these external and internal conflicts shattered basic assumptions of invulnerability and self-value. Many Kuwaitis probably experienced such stressful developments as narcissistic injuries.

According to the "just world" theory (Janoff-Bulman 1985), such shocking experiences are likely to increase the risk of PTSD. Breakdown of trust creates deep-seated insecurity and suspicion directed against friends and foes alike—and eventually hatred toward proven traitors. The effects of such human malice include fear, humiliation, hatred, helplessness, and hopelessness. Severe traumatization is likely to cause long-term psychopathology.

The Iraqi occupiers harassed not only the Kuwaitis themselves but also non-Kuwaitis with origins in countries that had joined the coalition against Iraq. Another group of non-Kuwaitis also suffered under the Iraqis: Bedouins. This group formed a large part of the lower ranks of the Kuwaiti police and army. Some fled to Saudi Arabia with their officers, separating from their families. Others were taken prisoner; because they were stateless, they found themselves in an extremely precarious situation.

As many as 70% of Kuwaiti families may have experienced separation from one another during the 7-month occupation. Of the approximately 400,000–450,000 Kuwaitis who were in the country at the beginning of the occupation, perhaps 250,000 escaped between August 2, 1990, and February 26, 1991. Only 47.3% of the respondents in the epidemiological survey had remained in Kuwait for the entire 7 months (Al-Hammadi et al. 1993).

Those remaining in Kuwait faced a constant threat of danger. They could never feel quite safe. Iraqi soldiers and security forces made death threats indiscriminately. Life became very unpredictable. Of Kuwaitis who were in the country at the time of the invasion, 55%— most of them women—went into hiding for 3 days or more (Al-Hammadi et al. 1993).

Iraqization. In late August 1990, as part of Iraq's plan to make Kuwait its 19th province, the occupiers removed the national symbols of Kuwait and punished anyone who attempted to display them. Automobile license plates, for example, had to be changed to Iraqi license plates. Kuwaiti citizens held out against this development, but a large proportion of Palestinian residents complied; Kuwaitis regarded this attitude as collaboration with the enemy.

Most teachers were Palestinians; all were ordered to teach the Iraqi version of the invasion. Kuwaitis therefore stopped sending their children to school, keeping them indoors for months for safety reasons. Most non-Kuwaitis, however, continued to send their children to school, which Kuwaiti citizens perceived as another sign of collaboration.

The Iraqi occupation forces issued decrees to set fire to and destroy the residence of anyone who possessed the picture of Kuwait's emir or prime minister or displayed the Kuwaiti national flag. When Iraqi soldiers were killed, the whole block where they died would be set on fire and destroyed. The Iraqis also imposed a curfew from dusk until dawn.

Thus, deprivation and loss of personal and national identity were prominent stressors for the Kuwaitis. In the face of this Iraqi harassment, many Kuwaitis escaped. During this period, numerous accounts of escapes through the desert, robberies and acts of violence en route, and deaths from various causes appeared.

The capacity to cope with severe stress (Antonovsky 1979) requires that the stressor be comprehensible, manageable, and meaningful. In this respect, the Kuwaiti situation was extremely problematic, especially for Kuwaiti citizens who could not escape. Societal values such as national identity, national cohesiveness, appreciation of freedom, and willingness to make sacrifices are important for a nation's tolerance of severe stress. In spite of such resilience factors, however, the war clearly had a terrifying affect on the people of Kuwait.

Sexual assault. Kuwaitis were greatly concerned about rape and other forms of sexual violence during the occupation. Cultural factors make rape an especially severe psychic trauma in a Moslem country. Because abortion and adoption arrangements for infants of unwanted pregnancies are unacceptable, unwanted pregnancy secondary to rape is even more difficult.

Health professionals reported that women who had been raped began to ask for help in the immediate wake of the invasion in August 1990. The number of cases increased with more terror-inducing behavior by the occupation forces, especially after October 1990.

The actual number of rape victims is not known, even approximately. Physicians at one of Kuwait's six public hospitals reported that they examined and treated 60 cases during the occupation. These cases, however, may represent only a small fraction of individuals actually affected. In the epidemiological survey, the majority of respondents who reported rapes were men (Al-Hammadi et al. 1993).

The Iraqis perpetrated individual and group rape, including heterosexual and homosexual rape. Kuwaitis also reported sadistic rape involving bodily mutilation and sometimes murder. These rapes sometimes took place in the presence of the victim's family members; in some instances, entire families were raped. In addition to committing rape as an act of torture and terror, the Iraqis used rape as a method to insult and humiliate families, as well as the entire nation.

Not unexpectedly, health professionals (including gynecologists, psychiatrists, psychologists, and others) reported that female patients who had been raped were emotionally distressed and anxious and needed substantial support. Suicidal thoughts and acts were common; many victims developed concentration problems, fear of men and sexuality, depression, and social withdrawal. Victims' reluctance to speak about the rape increased over time.

Children.   A preliminary report based on a study of 2,422 school children (ages 7–17 years) who had been in Kuwait during all or part of the occupation found that the majority of the sample had witnessed arrests (Elisa and Nofel 1993). In addition, 14% witnessed someone being injured or killed, and 26% had seen a dead body. Nearly 7% had been physically harmed, and 38% reported having experienced fear for their lives. Children ages 11–17 years had experienced more traumas than younger children.

Resistance.   Even in the first days of the occupation, many Kuwaitis experienced the hatred that Iraqi soldiers harbored against them. Mass arrests of Kuwaiti military personnel began immediately after the invasion; many of these detainees were transported to Iraq. Already on August 8, 1990, Kuwaiti women and their children demonstrated in the streets against the invaders. The Iraqis met this demonstration with gunfire; one person was killed and a number were wounded.

Kuwaitis often were punished or threatened with death even for minor infractions (e.g., having Kuwaiti money). Although active resistance was not necessary to elicit life-threatening confrontations, the Iraqis severely punished such activities; this punishment included harsh reprisals.

The occupiers systematically used the threat of execution to obtain information about resistance fighters. The Iraqi forces often carried out summary execution, torture, and rape in front of family members as an act of collective punishment and deterrence. Severe torture often was followed by execution; the body may have been left in front of the victim's house for days, with the family forbidden to remove and bury it—thus violating important religious obligations. The Iraqis tortured and executed children as well as adults—sometimes parents and children together.

Torture sometimes involved crude techniques, such as progressively cutting off parts of the body. Moreover, in contrast with some Nazi methods—for example, the "night and fog" system, which aimed at maximizing fear through uncertainty about what had happened to victims—the Iraqis apparently did not attempt to cover up their atrocities in Kuwait. Their actions may have been part of a deliberate campaign to terrorize the population.

The Iraqis also attempted to force Kuwaitis to abuse other Kuwaitis, even family members.

Ninety-four percent of Kuwaitis who reported torture were men; men also constituted the vast majority of Kuwaitis who reported having been taken hostage or detained for more than 3 days. More than 10% of adult Kuwaiti men reported each of these psychological stressors (Al-Hammadi et al. 1993).

The epidemiological survey (Al-Hammadi et al. 1993) found that 40% of Kuwaiti men and women had personally witnessed violence, and 40% of the families of martyrs had witnessed the death of their family member. Although the actual number of Kuwaitis killed probably was far lower than the early estimate of approximately 7,000, most Kuwaitis could report that a family member had been killed or was missing; the large size of extended Kuwaiti families helps to explain this phenomenon. According to hospital records, the Iraqis inflicted 2,552 war injuries; this number, however, surely is an underestimate because many Kuwaitis sought treatment elsewhere, and doctors often tried not to register such cases in hospital records.

Breakdown of services. Health services deteriorated significantly during the occupation. Inpatient and outpatient services were reduced; the numbers of medical staff declined dramatically because of transport and safety problems, as well as the fact that many health care workers escaped the country. As a result, deaths increased, particularly among the most vulnerable patients (e.g., mentally retarded individuals). One institution reported that 50% of the 200 patients who were not evacuated by their relatives died. Approximately 10% of patients remaining in the only psychiatric hospital in Kuwait died.

This mortality rate is typical of wartime occupations; two- to threefold increases in mortality are common. The reduced admission rates reported by the psychiatric hospital also are typical for war, partly reflecting reduced capacity for services and partly indicating an increased willingness of families to care for their ill members.

The country also experienced breakdowns in garbage collection, food distribution, and public transportation. In the last weeks of the occupation, electricity and water supplies were cut off.

Throughout the occupation, the Iraqis looted homes and confiscated cars owned by Kuwaitis and coalition nationals. Many facilities were stripped of all furniture and equipment. Such measures increased toward the end of the occupation. However, some sections of Kuwait City reported relatively few Iraqi soldiers and few incidents of looting.

Motivational forces.   The factors that led to the formation of the anti-Iraq military coalition also provided the strongest motivation for Kuwaitis. The survival strategies of fight and flight, along with hiding, appeared quickly in occupied Kuwait; very few Kuwaitis seem to have surrendered. In particular, the absence of traitors and collaborators among Kuwaiti citizens was significant. A relatively large portion of the proportion succeeded in fleeing.

Fear, grief, anger, and despair were widespread and often constant reactions during the occupation. Terror—particularly the pervasive fear of sexual assaults and other threats—induced a state of constant vigilance. This vigilance led to many symptoms of stress including lack of sleep; parents struggled to protect and control their children.

The most frequent concerns during the occupation related to family safety and Kuwait's future (Al-Hammadi et al. 1993). Kuwaitis also reported widespread concerns about threats of death, rape, and unprovoked searches; looting and destruction; torture; fear of the future; and the loss of Kuwait's identity. Many Kuwaiti nationals were driven into their houses and did not leave because of the unsafe situation. To some extent, they had to rely on non-Kuwaitis to bring them food and other necessities. This reliance led to mixed feelings: gratitude, tempered at times by feelings that they were being exploited.

The relative absence of health services led to a reduction in their use. Alcohol and drug use, however, increased; the Iraqi army lifted the traditional ban on alcohol, probably as a way of demoralizing the population. Within institutions, only severely mentally retarded persons did not show signs of stress. Psychiatric patients generally became easier to handle for the few personnel who could work. Psychoses precipitated by specific war traumas were largely left in the hands of the occupying forces and were not referred to the health services for treatment. Health workers observed that the occupation even had positive effects on some individuals who previously had suffered from neurotic symptoms. Instances of improved family attitudes toward persons with mental problems also were reported.

Among traditional and informal support systems, *Diwaniyas* played an important role in helping Kuwaitis to cope with the stress of the occupation. Strangely, the occupying forces did not prohibit this unique Kuwaiti social custom—in which one man invites a circle of men and boys he trusts to an informal meeting in his house. In addition to providing social support, *Diwaniyas* enabled Kuwaitis to exchange sensitive information.

In the last weeks of the occupation—during the intensive coalition bombing of Iraq—the general situation in the occupied country deteriorated dramatically, while Kuwaiti hopes for liberation rose. Looting and deliberate destruction of property by the Iraqis intensified. At this time, several thousand Kuwaitis—mainly young men—were taken hostage and deported to Iraq, reportedly to be used as "human shields." An undisclosed number of these Kuwaitis probably perished in the Iraqi convoys that were destroyed while fleeing the allied onslaught.

Liberation

In the face of Operation Desert Storm, the Iraqi army fled Kuwait, putting up little resistance; as a result, physical destruction and loss of life were limited during the liberation. Joy and relief were the dominant psychological reactions among Kuwaitis during the liberation phase. Nevertheless, the fact that Saddam Hussein was still in power in Iraq, continuing to express threats about annexing Kuwait, added to Kuwaiti feelings of insecurity.

Most of the Kuwaitis who had been out of the country at the time of the invasion, or had subsequently escaped, returned to find their properties vandalized and looted. This destruction caused major distress for some, but many considered such circumstances to be minor compared with more tragic events that befallen them and their family members.

Returning Kuwaitis encountered many physical hardships including the destruction of the oil wells (most of which were on fire). This Iraqi sabotage represented a loss of national resources: much of Kuwait's future income was burning.

The oil fires also caused a major environmental disaster; the pollution of air and water provided a major additional stress including prolonged concern for children. Toxic gases caused an increase of respiratory, allergic, skin, and coronary symptoms. This pollution forced many Kuwaitis to stay indoors. Particles in the polluted air also carried an unknown long-term risk for the development of cancers.

Physicians frequently attributed psychic manifestations of posttraumatic stress and anxiety syndrome to the air contamination, consistent with environmental stress syndrome. The lesser stigma of somatic, as compared with psychological, symptoms probably contributed to this explanation for apparently strange behavior among some Kuwaitis. Kuwaitis who had endured the occupation, however, seemed to feel less threatened by the pollution. Their sense of relief after having survived the ordeal may have played a part in this response.

The many types and large quantities of mines left in the desert and on the beaches provided a constant reminder that danger was still present. The air pollution and mines also restricted Kuwaitis' freedom of movement, affecting their basic feeling of independence.

Kuwaiti civil authority was absent in the immediate postliberation period, and some groups of Kuwaitis took advantage of the situation to express their pent-up hatred and frustration against collaborators. At times, suspicion of collaboration extended to all persons whose countries of origin did not support the anti-Iraq coalition. Unfortunately, this attitude led some Kuwaitis to commit acts that repeated the treatment they had suffered at the hands of their occupiers. Thus, Kuwaitis acted out the cycle of violence.

Postwar Period

As a result of the war, the Kuwaiti government took a major decision to reduce its reliance on imported labor. This policy was enforced quickly; the new policy, coupled with harassment of non-Kuwaitis because of actual or suspected collaboration, led a large number of guest workers to leave the country.

As a result of this development, up to 7,000 families with a Kuwaiti mother and a non-Kuwaiti father—or a father whose country of origin supported Iraq during the war—faced a stressful dilemma. The fathers could not return to Kuwait, or, if they were already in the country, they had to leave. Thus, mothers and children were forced to separate from their husbands and fathers or leave their home country. Stressful events such as these present well-known psychiatric risk factors.

In 1991, following the liberation, 33 Kuwaitis died from injuries caused by mines and ammunition; 24 Kuwaitis (mostly children and adolescents) died from this cause in 1992. As of mid-February 1993, a total of 1,243 Kuwaitis had suffered such war-related injuries.

Psychiatric Disturbances

War trauma affected behavior and emotions. After the liberation, Kuwaitis exhibited decreased respect for law and authority, especially among young people. Directors of institutions for juvenile delinquents (ages 7–17 years) reported an increase in crime; delinquent acts seemed to be more violent than before the war. A systematic study (Al-Hammadi et al. 1993) subsequently supported this anecdotal evidence.

Many Kuwaitis described typical posttraumatic stress reactions. Teachers noted reduced concentration in school children and reported a significant number of new cases of school phobia, probably secondary to the fact that schools were used by the Iraqis as places for torture. Elisa and Nofel (1993) found that girls ages 11–17 years exhibited more severe PTSD than the rest of the population; 11% were classified as severe PTSD and 0.4% as very severe.

Teachers also reported more fighting among school children, more questioning of teacher authority, and even threats directed at teachers, some involving firearms. Such behavior would have been unheard of previously. Increased divorce rates after the liberation probably were caused largely by problems related to intermarriage with non-Kuwaiti nationalities. Sexual traumatization of a spouse also may have been a factor in some divorces.

Rape

The long-term psychosocial consequences of rape persisted in the postoccupation period. Sexual torture and rape cause feelings of stigma and shame; a statement by Kuwaiti leaders that acknowledged raped men and women as martyrs—citizens who had paid a high price for the nation's occupation—would have helped.

Kuwaiti cultural traditions, however, were strong. Kuwaiti victims of unwitnessed rape often tried to keep the incident a secret from their families. Unfortunately, however, many instances of rape had been witnessed; in other cases, Kuwaitis surmised such assaults because they knew that women taken into custody frequently were raped. Because such traumatization endangered family honor, victims and their families dealt with the consequences silently. As a result, human support, which is crucial in the recovery process of rape victims, often was absent. Young unmarried women, bereft of their virginity, had serious problems regarding their prospects for future marriage.

Social Response to War Trauma

Kuwaiti society generally accepted psychic war traumatization; Kuwaitis also regarded psychological injuries as evidence of the Iraqis' cruelty. However, many young men felt that acknowledging posttraumatic stress reactions would be a sign of weakness that they did not want to admit to the still-threatening Iraqi aggressor.

After the war, family physicians at the primary health care center reported a general increase in requests for hypnosis and tranquilizers from their patients. A substantial proportion of patients—perhaps more than 30%—reported complaints that were colored, precipitated, exacerbated, or caused by war-related stress. Somatization was a frequent presentation. Strikingly, many patients expected immediate relief; nearly all of them expected (and received) medications for their ailments.

Kuwaiti Torture Victims and Prisoners of War

Predictably, the incidence of PTSD and other psychiatric disorders after the war and occupation was highest among victims of torture and prisoners of war (many of whom also suffered torture). Early in 1992, the Al-Riggae Specialist Center for Treatment of War Related Victims began to register persons who sought help for such problems. This center was founded by the Kuwaiti Ministry of Public Health and modeled on a similar center established by the International Rehabilitation Council for Torture Victims; it was the first rehabilitation center for torture survivors in an Arab country.

Stæhr et al. (1993) reported on 250 patients treated at the Al-Riggae Center during its first 7 months of operation. Of these patients, three-fourths of the children ($N = 57$) received a psychiatric diagnosis (primarily PTSD). Approximately 64% of the adult patients were torture survivors, and 35% were victims of human rights violations; only 1% had sought help because they were disabled by mine or ammunition explosions. These findings support an earlier report from the United Nations Commission on Human Rights (1992).

All of the torture survivors had been exposed to psychological torture; three-quarters also had experienced physical torture. One-third had been imprisoned outside Kuwait. Of the torture survivors, 76% received a psychiatric diagnosis. Of these, 64% had PTSD as their primary diagnosis, and 22% had depression. As many as 90% of the former POWs suffered from PTSD. Judged from scores on the 10-item Post-Traumatic Symptom Scale (Weisæth 1989), the PTSD conditions were severe.

Relief and recognition by an official government clinic appeared to be a major factor affecting the wish and need for further treatment. Many patients, however, dropped out of psychotherapy because of difficulties in following the timetable of appointments.

National Epidemiological Study

The Al-Riggae study (Al-Hammadi et al. 1993) hoped to define the relationship between the different types and levels of trauma experienced by families during the occupation and their posttraumatic psychological symptoms 2 1/2 years after the liberation. For this study, a group of health workers who had received 2 weeks of training interviewed a representative national sample of 566 families ($N = 2,856$ individuals). They collected data on traumatic stress exposures and self-report symptom inventories: the Hopkins Symptom Checklist-25 (HSCL-25), a PTSD scale, and the Impact of Event Scale (IES) (Horowitz et al. 1979). The investigators did not carry out clinical diagnostic interviews, however.

The researchers chose an IES total score of 39.5 as the cutoff point to identify a case of PTSD. The study's point prevalences of PTSD must be considered preliminary, however. No data were available on prewar baseline prevalences of PTSD or other psychiatric disorders in Kuwait; as a result, precise pre- and postwar comparisons were impossible. However, the war content of IES items increases the specific relationship between PTSD and war trauma to some extent.

The study excluded children younger than 6 years. Kuwaitis represented 94% of the sample; the study therefore includes insufficient data on minority groups. The investigators compared the random sample with three other groups from the Kuwaiti population: families of martyrs, of missing POWs, and of Kuwaitis who were injured during the occupation.

The distribution of HSCL-25 and IES scores indicated that a significant majority of people covered by categories of war trauma established by the United Nations Compensation Commission for Kuwait (UNCC) experienced distressing symptoms. Subjects exhibited a variety of typical posttraumatic stress reactions; high scores of clinical severity were compatible with PTSD. The IES data demonstrated that this distress was specifically related to the Iraqi occupation. Almost half of the adults (48.5%) scored above the cutoff point on the HSCL-25; 27.1% were above the IES cutoff point, and 24.5% had high scores on the PTSD scale. Thus, about one in four subjects exhibited PTSD, according to the self-reported scales. (Pearson correlation between the scales was highly significant.)

Women and young adults had a higher rate of PTSD, presumably because they had been more active during the occupation. In addition, 44% of the children exhibited behavioral disturbances such as conduct disorders; 16.8% were diagnosed with PTSD. Among adult family members of martyrs, POWs, and injured persons, the prevalences of PTSD (judged solely by IES score) were 42.5%, 32.7%, and 33.7%, respectively.

Neither the levels of distress nor PTSD differed noticeably among subjects within the UNCC war trauma categories. However, the numbers of victims in some categories (death of family member, injured, sexual assault) constituted too small a basis for statistical comparisons of PTSD rates. The mean PTSD prevalence among people in the UNCC war trauma categories was 34.5%—somewhat higher than the random sample average.

International Ex-Hostages

Approximately 1,200 British citizens (among other nationalities) were held hostage during the Iraqi occupation of Kuwait. Soon after their release, Easton and Turner (1991) estimated that 47% of these British hostages had suffered physical health deterioration and 21% had PTSD. Swedish hostages, who were exposed to lesser threat than the British, had relatively few problems after their release (Lundin and Ohlsson 1992).

Positive Aftereffects

Despite the distress and suffering experienced by Kuwaitis during the invasion, occupation, and liberation, some signs of positive outcomes also have appeared:

• An increased sense of cohesion in social networks where people learned to trust one another
• An increased sense of national identity among Kuwaitis who were abroad and particularly in those who remained
• An increased feeling of responsibility for the rehabilitation of the country and its future development.

COMPENSATION TO VICTIMS OF THE GULF WAR

Compensation for cruel, inhumane, or degrading treatment or punishment generally includes redress (i.e., moral assistance to victims, including victims' exemption from possible false accusations and just punishment of perpetrators), financial compensation, and treatment and rehabilitation of physical and psychological health problems. Iraq has not offered any redress, so the latter two types of compensation are the only forms available.

The United Nations Security Council established the UNCC after the war to facilitate such compensation. The UNCC represented the first effort by the United Nations to make an aggressor nation pay economic compensation for losses and damages from an invasion and occupation. Previous compensation schemes had involved bilateral arrangements between the aggressor and victim nations.

The UNCC proposed to award compensation for exposure to stressful war experiences, as well as for physical and psychological injuries (UNCC 1994). For smaller claims, the UNCC allowed claimants to seek compensation by establishing that they had experienced certain types of trauma during the war, without having to document the existence of specific patterns of distress. The premise for this practice was that mental pain and anguish would have a strong association with any of these traumas. The UNCC established five categories of war trauma:

A. Loss of spouse, child, or parent by death
B. Serious personal injury
C. Sexual assault or aggravated assault or torture
D. Witnessing the intentional infliction of any of these events (A, B, C) on a spouse, child, or parent
E. Having been taken hostage or illegally detained for more than 3 days with manifestly well-founded fear for one's life or fear of being taken hostage or illegally detained.

Some abuses, such as torture, usually cause serious injury and extend over long periods. For such cases, the UNCC determined that a claim under one category would provide grounds for a claim under another category.

The UNCC adopted ceilings rather than fixed amounts of compensation. Mental pain and anguish claims, for example, were limited to $100,000. The UNCC commissioners and Secretariat were empowered to consider modifying factors for each of the trauma categories.

The following aggravating factors would entitle a claimant in category A (death of spouse, child, or parent) to compensation at the highest amount:

• The claimant was younger than 21 years old and had lost both parents.
• The claimant was younger than 21 years old and had lost his or her only parent.
• The death of the claimants' family member occurred as a result of cruel, inhumane, or degrading treatment (e.g., death as a result of torture, execution, sexual assault, or being held as a "human shield").

Other aggravating factors that would justify an increase in the amount of compensation from a minimum lump-sum amount included multiple losses or one or more of the following:

- Deliberate actions leading to the death of the claimant's family member
- Degrading burial or other improper treatment of the deceased family member's body (e.g., no burial, family members not present, corpse not buried in accordance with the claimant's or deceased's religious practice or cultural expectations)
- Enforced period of time-lapse between death and burial
- Nonrecovery of a deceased family member's body
- Loss of an only child
- Loss of primary family support earner
- Death of a family member in which lack of medical care caused by the occupation of Kuwait contributed.

Mental Pain and Anguish

The UNCC recognized mental disorders within the category of serious personal injuries (category B). It determined that mental disorders should be assessed in terms of the International Classification of Diseases, Tenth Revision (ICD 10) (WHO 1991).

The UNCC provided compensation for mental pain and anguish on the basis of evidence that the situation described actually occurred. Claims submitted by individuals of many nationalities and collected by the UNCC reflected various levels of documentary evidence. Victims from poor countries with less developed health services often have less well-documented mental health problems. Because information concerning victims' cultures, personalities, and previous life experiences—which properly could be used in an assessment only on a case-by-case basis—usually was not included in the claims.

DISCUSSION

The major psychological stressors during the war in Kuwait—as assessed by the postwar WHO mission (WHO 1992)—related to physical injury, wounds, illnesses, and hardships; threats of death and threats to the safety of family members including conditions of uncertainty and helplessness; loss of loved ones; attack on human dignity and freedom; denial of personal and national identity; and witnessing horror and grotesque actions and the result of cruelties. Such stressors are likely to cause PTSD and other conditions in exposed subjects, and psychiatrists can safely predict that a wide range of war-related psychosocial problems will manifest themselves in the future.

Subsequent research supports predictions made by the WHO team. The national epidemiological study carried out 2 $^1/_2$ years after the end of the war (Al-Hammadi et al. 1993) represents an important investigation of the effects of trauma because of the quality of the sample and the range of outcome measures; no known previous research had examined a situation comparable with the occupation of Kuwait. Although aspects of the investigation's methodology may be subject to criticism (e.g., McFarlane 1993), the study clearly demonstrated a range of psychological symptoms among the civilian population of Kuwait that can be explained only by the war experience, rather than the prior existence of psychiatric disorders in the Kuwaiti population. The study reported levels of symptomatic distress that were significantly greater than—and different from—those found in nontraumatized communities.

Although the epidemiological study did not address vulnerability factors, it did identify traumatic stressors. Kuwaitis exposed to specific war traumas reported more posttraumatic stress problems than those without such exposure, although the differences were small. Surprisingly, the differences among the various trauma groups also were surprisingly small. Previous research and clinical experience in traumatic stress casts doubt on the hypothesis that forced hiding for as short as 3 days would be likely to lead to the same long-term or serious consequences as events in the other trauma categories.

By all measures, psychological distress was significant in adult and child populations. The constant, pervasive feeling of real threat, over a considerable period of time, probably created an intense fear and sense of helplessness in most of the Kuwaiti population—subsequently leading to long-term effects. If the terror strategies of the occupying forces were the cause of these psychological effects, the entire population was victimized.

The Kuwaiti population probably was rather vulnerable to the types of war experiences to which they were exposed. The population was not prepared for war, either mentally or in any other way. Given the combined effect of vulnerability and severe war traumas, the war had a terrifying effect overall on large segments of the population.

Theoretically, stressful events such as arrest, imprisonment, and torture that result from active resistance might produce less post-traumatic psychopathology than that exhibited by more passive war victims. Resisting individuals' comprehension of such stress, as well as the "manageability" or control and the "meaningfulness" of the stress, may account for such findings (Antonovsky 1979). Active resistance fighters also tend to be more stress resilient and exhibit positive coping mechanisms for war stress.

One positive aspect of the UNCC's work was that compensation could be provided to victims at a relatively early date and thereby have a preventive effect. Psychiatrists can expect delayed reactions, however; long lasting health problems are likely to develop, and some victims of severe trauma may find their work capacity reduced or destroyed. Ideally, the compensation scheme should include a follow-up program.

The absence of prospective, longitudinal studies limits analysis regarding the course of psychological trauma syndromes over time. Investigators do not know whether acute and subacute war-related effects will disappear or become mitigated at expected rates. The "Saddam factor" might affect the Kuwaiti population: the aggressor and his followers still represent a continued threat, and the war may not really be over. Invasive reexperience of the traumatic stress situation is one characteristic symptom within the PTSD syndrome. As long as the basic threat has not been fully neutralized, a real traumatic stress situation may continue to prevail for the most severely traumatized individuals.

The war's massive, widespread effects also may have hidden the impact of particularly severe traumas. The most severe effects may manifest themselves in the long term. Investigators must conduct detailed, systematic follow-up studies of groups exposed to the most severe traumas and make diagnoses on the basis of structured clinical interviews; until they do, the rates of psychiatric disorders, including PTSD, must be considered merely suggestive.

CONCLUSION

Situations such as postwar Kuwait provide near-laboratory conditions for traumatic stress research. Investigators must intensify their efforts to study the concrete situation in Kuwait. More important, however, they must develop new scientific tools including theories, concepts, and measuring instruments to gain a deeper understanding of the long-term effects of war generally.

REFERENCES

Al-Hammadi A, Stæhr A, Behbehani J, et al: The Traumatic Events and Mental Health Consequences Resulting From the Iraqi Invasion and Occupation of Kuwait. Kuwait City, Public Authority of Compensation Resulting From Iraqi Aggression (PAAC), 1993

Antonovsky A: Health, Stress and Coping: New Perspectives on Mental and Physical Well-Being. San Francisco, CA, Jossey-Bass, 1979

Askevold F: War sailor syndrome. Psychother Psychosom 77:133–138, 1976/1977

Easton JA, Turner SW: Detention of British citizens as hostages in the Gulf: health, psychological, and family consequences. BMJ 303:1231–1234, 1991

Eitinger L: World War II in Norwegian psychiatric literature, in Wartime Medical Services. Edited by Lundberg JE, Otto U, Rydbeck B. Stockholm, Sweden, Försvarets forskningsanstalt, FOA, 1990, pp 413–425

Eitinger L, Strøm A: Mortality and Morbidity After Excessive Stress: A Follow-up Investigation of Norwegian Concentration Camp Survivors. Oslo, Norway, Universitetsforlaget, 1973

Elisa J, Nofel E: Screening for War Exposure and Post-Traumatic Stress Disorder Among Children in Kuwait, Age 7–17. Preliminary Report (in Arabic). Kuwait City, Ministry of Education, 1993

Giacaman R, Stoltenberg C, Weisæth L: Health, in Palestinian Society in Gaza, West Bank and Arab Jerusalem: A FAFO Survey of Living Conditions. Edited by Heiberg M, Øversen G. Oslo, Norway, Institute of Applied Social Science, 1993, pp 101–132

Green JD: Political reform and regime stability in the post-war Gulf. Terrorism 16:9–23, 1993

Horowitz M, Wilner N, Alvarez W: Impact of Event Scale: a measure of subjective distress. Psychosom Med 41:209–218, 1979

Janoff-Bulman R: The aftermath of victimization—rebuilding shattered assumptions, in Trauma and its Wake: The Study and Treatment of Posttraumatic Stress Disorder. New York, Brunner/Mazel, 1985, pp 15–36

Kaplan HI, Freedman AM, Sadock BJ (eds): Comprehensive Textbook of Psychiatry. Baltimore, MD, Williams & Wilkins, 1980

Keesing's Record of World Events. Cambridge, England, Longman Group, 1990

Keesing's Record of World Events. Cambridge, England, Longman Group, 1991

Lundin T, Ohlsson S: Early stress reactions among the Swedish hostages in Iraq 1990. Psychiatric Annals 23 (suppl):80–90, 1992

McFarlane AC: Main Report About the Validity of the Research Project "The Posttraumatic Events and Mental Health Consequences Resulting From the Invasion and Occupation of Kuwait." Geneva, Switzerland, World Health Organization, United Nations Compensation Commission, 1993

Ødegård Ø: The incidence of mental disease in Norway during World War II. Acta Psychiatrica Neurologica 29:333–353, 1954

Punamaki RL: Relationship between political violence and psychological responses among Palestinian women. Journal of Peace Research 27: 75–85, 1990

Stæhr AA, Bourisli B, Bøjholm S, et al: Description of selected groups of victims of war following the occupation and the late Gulf War. Kuwait City, Al-Riggae Specialist Center for Treatment of War-Related Victims, 1993

United Nations Commission on Human Rights: Situation of Human Rights in Occupied Kuwait. Geneva, Switzerland, United Nations Economic and Social Council, 1992

United Nations Compensation Commission (UNCC): Report of the Panel of Experts Appointed to Assist the United Nations Compensation Commission in Matters Concerning Compensation for Mental Pain and Anguish. Geneva, Switzerland, UNCC, 1994

Ursano RJ, Norwood AE (eds): Emotional Aftermath of the Persian Gulf War. Veterans, Families, Communities, and Nations. Washington, DC, American Psychiatric Press, 1996

Weisæth L: Torture of a Norwegian ship's crew: the torture, stress reactions and psychiatric after-effects. Acta Psychiatr Scand (suppl 355) 80:63–72, 1989

World Health Organization: International Classification of Diseases, 10th Revision. Geneva, Switzerland, World Health Organization, 1991

World Health Organization: Report of a WHO Mission on War-Related Mental Health Problems in Kuwait, October 1991. Geneva, Switzerland, World Health Organization, 1992

Chapter 7

Children of the Storm: A Study of School Children and Hurricane Andrew

Jon A. Shaw, M.D.

On August 24, 1992, Hurricane Andrew devastated south Miami, Florida, with winds up to 164 miles per hour. The storm
destroyed approximately 100,000 homes, apartments, and trailers
and left 85,000 people unemployed; 35 hurricane-related deaths were
reported. Although the storm's enormous destruction ended in
a matter of hours, the derivative effects of the disaster continued to
affect children and families, who had to adapt to the loss of a community. People who had lived in the community for years could not
find their way around. The geographical texture of the community
had been compromised with the loss of trees, road signs, and prominent architectural and natural markers. The 39 schools that were
hardest hit by Hurricane Andrew reported a 21% decline in the number of children registering for the new school year in September
1992—reflecting the flight of families from the hurricane area.

INITIAL RESPONSES

In the immediate aftermath of Hurricane Andrew, survivors were
preoccupied with the task of finding shelter, food, and water. Volunteer organizations responded with various degrees of rapidity to
establish shelters and food distribution sites and began to restore
logistical support systems. Yet these services were fragmented, un-
organized, and without central orchestration. The arrival of army
support units—with telecommunications systems, tent cities, public health capabilities, and food distribution—provided a much

needed infrastructure that was integral to the overall response to the community's needs.

Support providers focused primarily on life-support requirements and only secondarily on mental health needs. Nevertheless, they made efforts to provide crisis intervention services to the community and to provide information through the media regarding the storm's anticipated psychological effects on children. Volunteer mental health professionals provided crisis intervention services. A flyer called "Helping Children after Disaster"—patterned after the American Academy of Child and Adolescent Psychiatry's Facts for Families—was distributed throughout south Miami. Community meetings advertised through the media were held at churches and shopping malls (with little initial response).

One of the questions that arises after such a disaster is how to intervene most effectively on behalf of children and their families. In this chapter, I describe efforts by myself and my colleagues in the Division of Child and Adolescent Psychiatry at the University of Miami School of Medicine to respond to the disaster, using the schools as the predominant institution through which interventions were initiated. I discuss three initiatives: initial interventions in an elementary school in south Miami, focusing on work with teachers and children; a research study comparing children from an elementary school in the pathway of the storm with students from a school north of Miami that was spared the direct effects of Hurricane Andrew; and a multischool program that involved 88 crisis intervention specialists trained to intervene in schools most affected by Hurricane Andrew.

REDONDO ELEMENTARY SCHOOL

The first school intervention occurred at Redondo Elementary School in the Homestead area of south Miami. The school had been badly damaged in the storm: the roof leaked, and garbage cans had been distributed throughout the classrooms to catch rainwater; windows were broken; telephone communication, air conditioning, and other amenities such as running water were unavailable.

The principal invited me to meet with her and her teachers 3 days before the planned opening of school on September 14, 1992. She expressed concerns about her teachers, whom she described as demoralized and lacking initiative. She was particularly concerned about four or five teachers who were reluctant to share experiences, kept to themselves, and displayed a sense of frozen emotionality. She described other teachers as manifesting low frustration tolerance, heightened emotionality, feelings of anger, and depression.

I conducted a group discussion session with the teachers that focused on the context of disaster and its effects on children. In the debriefing exercise, I learned that 12 of the 25 teachers had lost their homes and had to find alternative shelter; five others had homes that were uninhabitable but had no other place to go. The teachers exhibited a general sense of helplessness and powerlessness including not knowing how to prioritize and begin to get their lives back together. Some teachers expressed fears of going crazy and feelings of despair, and several recounted stories of how they had been convinced they were going to die.

The teachers experienced considerable stress related not only to the hurricane per se but also to the ongoing process associated with the loss of home and community. The degree of demoralization, apathy, and perceived helplessness led my colleagues and me to focus first on assisting the teachers; we thereby hoped to facilitate their interactions with students.

To measure the teachers' posttraumatic symptomatology, we administered the Post-Traumatic Stress Disorder Research Inventory (PTSDRI) (Frederick 1985; Pynoos et al. 1987). In the initial assessment (September 11, 1992), 15% of the teachers exhibited mild posttraumatic symptomatology, and 81% manifested moderate to severe posttraumatic symptoms. We tracked the teachers' symptomatology throughout the remainder of the school year through repeated administrations of the PTSDRI (Table 7–1); the results indicated that posttraumatic symptomatology continued relatively unabated throughout the year. The assessment of March 24, 1993, occurred after a terrible storm with torrential rains and lightning that left many residents in the area panicked as they reexperienced all of the sights, sounds, fears, and anxieties associated with their exposure to Hurricane Andrew. Almost 60% of the teachers continued to experience moderate to severe posttraumatic symptoms 10 months after the hurricane. My colleagues and I believed that this continuing high

Table 7–1.   Posttraumatic stress symptomatology in elementary school teachers, Redondo Elementary School, Homestead, Florida

	September 11, 1992 (N = 26)		November 11, 1992 (N = 22)		March 24, 1993 (N = 27)		June 10, 1993 (N = 29)	
	n	%	n	%	n	%	n	%
Doubtful	1	3.8	2	9.1	2	7.4	4	13.8
Mild	4	15.4	5	22.7	6	22.2	8	27.6
Moderate	15	57.7	11	50.0	12	44.4	14	48.3
Severe	6	23.1	4	18.2	7	25.9	3	10.3
Very severe	0	0	0	0	0	0	0	0

Note.   Percentages may not add to 100% because of rounding.

prevalence of posttraumatic symptomatology was associated not only with continuing exposure to traumatic reminders but also with ongoing stressors, such as adversarial negotiations with insurance companies, contractors, and code inspectors as well as other stressors related to the slow, laborious recovery process.

Over the course of the school year, my colleagues and I met with the teachers in an ongoing group format and provided them with opportunities for individual sessions on an as-needed basis. We also met with students in all grades in the elementary school in classroom debriefing experiences. The format included a simple introduction about disaster and hurricanes and a brief description of normal psychological responses to scary experiences such as Hurricane Andrew.

In one exercise, we asked the children to draw a picture of the "worst moment of the hurricane"; their drawings invariably focused on funnel shaped and darkened clouds, broken trees, shattered windows, overturned cars, roofs blown off of homes, and continuing rain. The children frequently depicted tornado-like clouds as one-eyed or two-eyed monsters. The younger children associated "the eye" of the storm with a monster marching across the land and destroying homes.

We also gave each child a chance to tell his or her story to the class. This exercise provided the children with a normalizing experience, as well as an opportunity to express pent-up feelings and explore issues of blame and causality; it also helped us assess the children's cognitive distortions and offered us a way to identify children who were particularly stressed and needed more intense treatment interventions.

Some of the children were struggling not only with issues of posttraumatic symptomatology but also with psychological distress related to grief and bereavement and anxiety related to various types of separations. In one fifth-grade class, for example, 84% of the children said they were upset and afraid when they thought about the hurricane; 60% described sleep disturbances, 72% expressed fears that the hurricane would happen again, 40% spoke of nightmares, 56% talked of their fear of dying, and 52% spoke of avoiding thoughts and other reminders of the hurricane. One boy expressed his belief that the hurricane was a punishment for his having hit his brother, and a second boy related it to revenge for having killed insects.

POSTHURRICANE REACTIONS IN HIGH-IMPACT VERSUS LOW-IMPACT SCHOOLS

In the second school intervention, my colleagues and I studied the evolution of psychological effects of disaster among students at a *high-impact school* (HIS) directly in the pathway of Hurricane Andrew compared with students at a *low-impact school* (LIS), an elementary school north of Miami (as well as other schools in their respective districts).

Methods

In this study, my colleagues and I evaluated 106 children (56 boys, 50 girls) ages 6–11 years (mean age = 8.2, SD = 1.55). We studied a HIS ($n = 62$) in south Dade County and a LIS ($n = 44$) north of Miami. Table 7–2 presents various demographic variables for each school; the two schools were quite similar demographically.

Eight weeks after the hurricane, we administered Pynoos' PTSDRI—an instrument measuring the severity of exposure to the hurricane—to the children; also, the students' primary classroom teachers completed Achenbach's Teacher's Report Form (TRF) (Achenbach and Edelbrock 1983) for each child. Thirty-two weeks after the hurricane, we readministered the PTSDRI and the TRF to students at the HIS.

Table 7–2. Demographics of students at HIS and LIS

	HIS	LIS
Gender		
Males	37	19
Females	25	25
Racial/ethnic		
White	25	14
Black	10	11
Hispanic	24	14
Other	3	5
Primary language		
English	52	40
Spanish	8	3
Other	1	1
Grade*		
First	14	9
Second	20	8
Third	4	4
Fourth	16	17
Fifth	17	6
Live with mother		
Yes	56	43
No	5	1
Live with father		
Yes	42	29
No	19	1

Note.   HIS = high-impact school; LIS = low-impact school.
$*\chi^2 = 11.28, P < .05$.

We also obtained data on the frequency of 21 measures of covert and overt disruptive behavior from the Dade County Public Schools (DCPS) and analyzed these data by grading period for the prehurricane school year (1991–1992) and the posthurricane school year (1992–1993) for both the HIS and the LIS, as well as for their broader school regions—Region VI (HIS) and Region II (LIS). Measures of overt disruptive behavior included general disruptive behavior, defiance of school authority, disruption on the school bus, assault, theft, vandalism, battery on a student or staff member, fighting, robbery, continuous disruptive behavior, damaging school property, and aggravated assault. Measures of covert disruptive behavior included use of provocative language, cutting class, dress code violations, excessive unsatisfactory absences, presence in an unauthorized location, leaving class without permission, rude and discourteous behavior, excessive tardiness, and trespassing. We compared the proportion of students reported to the school district for these overt and covert disruptive behaviors for the year before and after the hurricane by grading period.

Results

The hurricane exposure instrument provided a method of determining the severity of exposure to the hurricane. As expected, students in the HIS had a significantly higher mean score (number of positive endorsements) (M = 6.0, SD = 2.1) than students in the LIS (M = 2.2, SD = 1.9) (t (115) = 10.51, P < .0001); Table 7–3 presents individual item endorsements for the HIS and the LIS with supporting χ^2 tests. The severity of exposure for students in the HIS is evident: 82% of the students had a window broken or door blown open; 57% had part of a roof blown away or caved in; 87% reported being scared that a loved one would be hurt or killed; 24% reported a pet hurt or killed; and 39% reported staying out of their home when the hurricane was over.

The great majority of students at both schools exhibited posttraumatic symptoms: 87% of the children at the HIS and 80% of the children at the LIS manifested at least moderate levels of posttraumatic symptomatology. The HIS had twice as many students in the severe category; however, the schools did not differ significantly in posttraumatic symptoms.

On the TRF, t tests indicated that LIS students demonstrated more psychopathology than HIS students. Boys at the HIS had significantly lower scores on the "unpopular" scale than boys at the LIS (P = .05); girls in the HIS exhibited significantly lower mean scores

Table 7–3. Hurricane damage exposure for HIS and LIS

Item	HIS (N = 62)		LIS (N = 44)		χ^2	P
	n	%	n	%		
Doors or windows break or come open?	51	82.3	5	11.4	51.91	<.0001
Roof blown away or cave in?	35	56.5	2	4.5	30.52	<.0001
Did you get hurt?	3	4.8	1	2.3	0.47	NS
Did anyone with you get hurt?	10	16.1	0	0	7.84	.005
Were you scared that a loved one would be hurt/killed?	54	87.1	29	65.9	6.80	.009
Did you see anyone get hurt?	7	11.3	2	4.5	1.51	NS
Was anyone with you very scared?	54	87.1	30	68.2	5.60	.018
Did you get wet from rain/seawater?	36	58.0	6	13.6	21.23	<.0001
Went outside because of damage to home?	8	12.9	1	2.3	3.74	<.053
Did a pet get hurt or die?	15	24.2	2	4.5	7.38	.007
Stay out of your home after the hurricane?	24	38.7	4	9.1	11.96	.001
Are you still out of your home?	12	19.4	0	0	9.60	.002
Did a grownup lose his/ her job?	15	24.2	3	6.8	5.51	.019
Did you lose anything important?	25	40.3	11	25.0	2.69	NS
Did your family get separated for awhile?	5	8.1	1	2.3	1.62	NS
Do you feel safe since the hurricane? ("No" responses)	9	14.5	2	4.5	2.75	NS
Trouble getting food or water?	24	38.7	14	31.8	0.53	NS

Note. N = 106. HIS = high-impact school; LIS = low-impact school; NS = not significant.

on internalizing ($P < .01$), externalizing ($P < .05$), anxious ($P < .01$), unpopular ($P < .01$), self-destructive ($P < .05$), and aggressive ($P < .05$) than girls in the LIS (Table 7–4). At 32 weeks posthurricane, repeat PTSDRI measures on children in the HIS demonstrated a significant reduction in PTSDRI symptomatology: X ($4, N = 64) = 17.3$, $P < .005$ (Figure 7–1).

Next we compared the proportion of students reported to DCPS for overt and covert disruptive behavior for the two specific schools, as well as for the educational regions where the HIS (Region VI) and the LIS (Region II) are located, for each grading period for the school years before and after the hurricane. School-based disruptive behavior (both overt and covert) showed a marked decrease ($P < .0001$) in prevalence for the grading period immediately following the hurricane in Region VI (Figure 7–2) but a marked increase ($P < .0001$) in Region II compared with the school year preceding the hurricane (Figure 7–3). The prevalence of overt behavior in Region VI returned to the previous year's level by the second grading period; covert behavior, however, rose significantly ($P < .0001$) above the previous year's levels.

The school-level data revealed a simpler but similar trend. In the first and second grading periods, the HIS had a significant decrease in overt and covert disruptive behaviors ($P < .05$). The third grading period showed a significant increase in overt behavior ($P < .01$), while

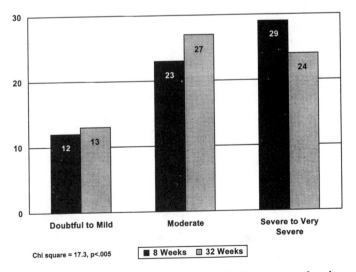

Figure 7–1. PTSDRI symptomatology in high-impact school.

Table 7–4. Means and standard deviations on teacher report form, by school and gender

| | Boys | | | | Girls | | | |
| | HIS | | LIS | | HIS | | LIS | |
	Mean	SD	Mean	SD	Mean	SD	Mean	SD
Internalizing	1.92	2.76	4.31	5.65	2.92	5.20	9.15	8.19
Externalizing	10.27	13.65	17.38	18.42	6.64	8.63	16.85	20.13
Anxious	0.92	1.67	2.50	3.33	1.56	3.37	6.20	5.52
Socially withdrawn	1.00	1.41	1.81	2.99	1.36	2.53	2.95	3.49
Unpopular	0.70	1.05	1.75	1.81	0.76	1.30	4.30	4.74
Self-destructive	0.41	0.86	0.56	0.73	0.28	0.54	1.20	1.64
Obsessive-compulsive	0.77	1.06	1.13	1.36	0.08	0.28	0.30	0.73
Inattentive	4.68	5.32	7.69	7.52	3.96	6.23	6.60	8.56
Nervous-overactive	0.81	1.17	1.38	1.41	1.00	1.44	1.80	1.99
Aggressive	4.78	8.89	8.32	11.02	1.68	2.30	8.45	11.51

Note. HIS = high-impact school; LIS = low-impact school; SD = standard deviation.

Relative Risk

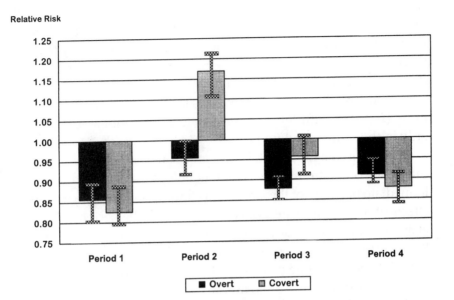

Figure 7–2. Overt and covert disruptive behavior for posthurricane school year, by grading period, Region VI.

Relative Risk

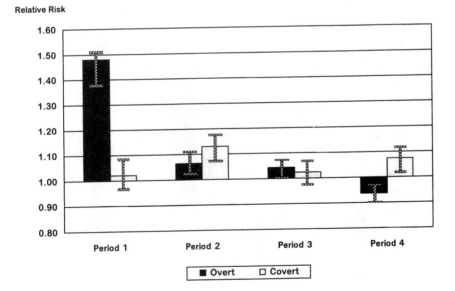

Figure 7–3. Overt and covert disruptive behavior for posthurricane school year, by grading period, Region II.

covert behavior returned to the preceding year's level; in the fourth grading period, the levels of overt behavior returned to the preceding year's levels, but covert behavior decreased significantly ($P \leq .05$) (Figure 7–4). The trends in the LIS, however, look very different (Figure 7–5). The LIS had a significant increase in the likelihood of overt and covert disruptive behaviors for the first three grading periods ($P < .05$), with levels returning to the previous year's levels only in the fourth grading period.

Children in the LIS had the same prevalence of mild and moderate categories of posttraumatic symptomatology as did children in the immediate pathway of the storm. This finding suggests the important effects of media exposure, anticipatory anxiety, the peripheral impact of the storm, and initial uncertainty about where the storm would strike; Kiser et al. (1993) described the effects of anticipatory anxiety in initiating mild and moderate posttraumatic symptomatology in a group of school children who were told that an earthquake would occur (which, in fact, never happened). Following Hurricane Andrew, children in the HIS were twice as likely to have severe to very severe symptoms—confirming that psychological distress is correlated with proximity to the zone of impact.

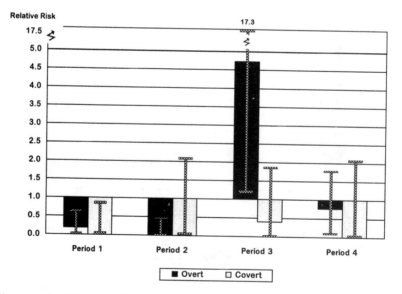

Figure 7–4.   Overt and covert disruptive behavior for posthurricane school year, by grading period, high-impact school.

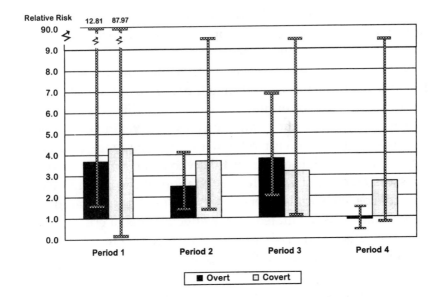

Figure 7–5. Overt and covert disruptive behavior for posthurricane school year, by grading period, low-impact school.

In the immediate aftermath of the hurricane, children in the HIS manifested reduced indices of psychopathology on the TRF compared with those in the LIS. The HIS and the other 38 schools in Region VI reported significantly reduced overt and covert disruptive behavior compared with the previous school year, the LIS, and the other 36 schools in Region II. My colleagues and I believe that the decrease in non-PTSDRI emotional and behavioral problems was related to generic, shock-like, numbing effects in the immediate aftermath of the hurricane that dampened behavioral responses to the disaster.

The initial decline in non-PTSDRI emotional and disruptive behaviors in the HIS and its larger educational area (Region VI) was followed by a rebound effect and then a relatively quick return to normalcy. However, there was an increase in overt and covert disruptive behaviors and apparently increased levels of psychopathology (as measured by the TRF) at the LIS and its larger school region (Region II) in the first grading period after the hurricane. These increases probably were partially related to the flight of refugees from south Dade County, a 6% increase in the school population in

Region II, a 13% increase in the student population at the LIS, and Region II's relative scarcity of support services (which were increasingly focused on the hurricane area).

My colleagues and I speculate that the initial high levels of PTSDRI symptomatology reflected the *event trauma* (i.e., Hurricane Andrew), and the continuing high levels of PTSDRI symptomatology at 32 weeks and the relative increase midyear in overt and covert disruptive behavior related to the emergence of a *process trauma*. The initial disaster was followed by an array of secondary stressors associated with the devastation of the community and multiple psychosocial adversities. We believe that the rapid return to normalcy was facilitated by the effectiveness of crisis intervention specialists and crisis mobile teams that were introduced in Region VI in November 1992.

CRISIS INTERVENTION SPECIALISTS

Our third intervention involved an effort to use the county school system as a conduit for providing systematic mental health services to the community. This effort paralleled the ongoing research effort described earlier.

In fall 1992, DCPS asked the Division of Child and Adolescent Psychiatry to provide a training and supervisory experience for 88 new counseling and visiting teacher/school social work positions assigned to the school regions most affected by Hurricane Andrew. Sixty-eight of these crisis intervention specialists were assigned to specific schools to supplement intrinsic counseling services; the other 20 were divided into four crisis response teams whose mission was to visit schools within the catchment area on a regular basis and respond to specific crises emanating from specific schools.

With this mandate, my colleagues and I established a training program for school counselors and newly appointed crisis intervention specialists in the identification and treatment of posttraumatic stress symptomatology in children and adolescents. The first 2-day conference occurred November 3, 1992. This meeting included presentations concerning perspectives on community disaster, psychological responses of children and adolescents to disaster, the role of the school in disaster, and intervention strategies in the school setting.

The crisis intervention specialists were then divided into eight teams, each with a team leader from the faculty of the Division of Child and Adolescent Psychiatry. The teams met 2–3 hours every 2 weeks throughout the academic year; these meetings provided a training, supervisory, and consultation experience within which the crisis intervention specialists could present clinical cases, consultation and liaison problems, intervention and treatment issues, and their use of community resources. A presentation by the team leader at each session was an important part of the training experience. The teams addressed topics such as identification of posttraumatic symptomatology, treatment strategies, child and adolescent development, stress management techniques, grief and bereavement, suicidal behavior, depression in children and adolescents, disruptive behavior problems, uses of nonverbal modalities in therapy, consultation strategies, and crisis intervention strategies.

A second all-day conference in February 1993 emphasized other psychiatric sequelae associated with disaster. The participants increasingly recognized that, with the passage of time, the spectrum of psychological distress had changed; the new pattern reflected the enduring derivative effects of Hurricane Andrew: psychosocial adversity; increasing indices of social maladjustment; reported increases in child abuse; marital and family dysfunction; adversarial relations with insurance companies, contractors, and code inspectors; and the extraordinary slowness of the recovery and restorative phase.

My colleagues and I implemented a systematic review of the effectiveness of this training program by distributing itemized questionnaires to the various groups involved in the process: the school principals, school counselors assigned to the schools, and the crisis intervention specialists themselves. These instruments asked respondents to rate specific aspects of the program on a scale of 1–7 (1 = no or not at all, 7 = extremely well).

The 26 school principals in Region VI were uniformly positive about the training and effectiveness of the crisis intervention specialists in their schools. The principals judged the crisis intervention specialists to be well prepared to handle crisis situations and family interventions, assist school counselors, work cooperatively together, work with students in small groups, provide relief to teachers and staff, and handle the types of problems the students presented; the composite score for these indices was 6.3. The principals also strongly supported the efforts of the intervention specialists in their specific schools (composite score 6.8) and the region (6.4) and noted that they wanted the program to continue the next year (6.8). Other specific comments by the school principals included the following:

- Excellent job
- Continue to fund for 1993–1994
- Our intervention specialist has been effective in her role
- Excellent articulation with staff, students, and community
- The program has been a precious tool to assist our students
- You have the right job description, but we need someone of the same ethnicity
- A much needed program
- They need more extensive crisis intervention training
- I found the additional counseling help invaluable
- Provide additional training in the grieving process
- Members of the intervention team have fulfilled all requisites in an exemplary manner

The 21 school counselors from schools in Region VI were equally enthusiastic about the crisis intervention specialists who assisted them. The counselors reported that the crisis intervention specialists they observed were prepared to handle the types of problems that the students presented (composite score 5.8), prepared to handle crisis situations (6.4), prepared to handle family interventions (5.6), and prepared to work with the students in small groups (6.0). The school counselors were very supportive of the efforts of intervention specialists at their school (6.8) and in the region (6.6). The school counselors rated the overall effectiveness of the program as 6.3. Additional specific comments by the school counselors included the following:

- Important for both counselors and intervention specialists to know their roles
- More training dealing with parents would be useful
- Expand program for all schools
- Update each year
- Intervention specialists have done an excellent job
- More in-service training is need for crisis intervention specialists

- Emphasize communication and problem-solving skills
- The program should be continued next year
- The teams did not seem as effective as the individual specialist
- The intervention specialists have done an awful lot to decrease suspensions and increase attendance
- I highly recommend school on-site intervention specialists at each school next year
- Teams need training in working with diverse student populations

The crisis intervention specialists themselves also responded positively. Table 7–5 presents the responses of 54 crisis intervention specialists to questions regarding their training experience and self-reported effectiveness.

DISCUSSION

The psychological effects of disastrous events on children has emerged as a focus of study (Bloch et al. 1956; Burke et al. 1986; Green et al. 1991; Kiser et al. 1993; Newman 1976; Pynoos et al. 1987; Terr 1981, 1983). Terr (1991) noted the important role of psychic trauma as a crucial etiological factor in the development of many serious psychiatric disorders of childhood and adulthood. Studies of children after natural disaster have consistently demonstrated a spectrum of posttraumatic symptoms including trauma-specific fears; fears of recurrence; anxiety; intrusive recollection of images and perceptions of the traumatic event; posttraumatic play; behavioral reenactments; regressive behavior; somatic ills; avoidance of traumatic reminders; behavioral and school problems; and changed attitudes about the self, the world, and the future.

The context of each disaster, the identified population, and the postdisaster time frame determine the development and implementation of mental health services to help children suffering from the psychological consequences of the disaster (Cohen 1988). In times of crisis, logistical and medical support systems often become overwhelmed and focus their efforts on survival issues. The interventions described in this chapter focused on the schools as the most expeditious and effective conduit through which to provide prevention/intervention programs for children who are the victims of community disaster. Under such circumstances, concerns for the

Table 7–5. Intervention specialists questionnaire

Index	Composite score
The full day training sessions provided clinical interventions that were helpful when working with the children.	5.4
The small training group meetings have been helpful.	6.3
The didactic teaching in the small group meetings is clinically useful when working with the children.	6.3
The case presentations/discussions have facilitated my interventions with the children.	6.0
The small group sessions provide an opportunity to share the problems and frustrations of being an intervention specialist.	6.7
The small group meetings are helpful in dealing with the problems of working within the school system.	6.2
The small group sessions encourage group participation and involvement.	6.6
The group leaders are knowledgeable and interesting.	6.5
My efforts have been appreciated by the regular counselors.	6.0
My efforts have been appreciated by the students.	6.5
My efforts have been appreciated by the parents.	6.2
The training has adequately prepared me to work with students in the role of intervention specialist.	6.0
The training has adequately prepared me to handle crisis situations.	5.8
The training has adequately prepared me to handle family interventions.	5.1
I receive adequate support from the counselor in my school.	5.8
I receive adequate support from the crisis teams.	5.8

Note. $N = 54$.

well-being of children must be addressed through the rapid reopening of schools. The reestablishment of this social structure is the natural medium to begin delivering services to child victims.

Implementing a school-based intervention strategy is a delicate task; it requires sensitive interaction with a complex, multilayered bureaucracy that is very concerned with boundaries and preroga-tives and strives to be independent of outside influences. Necessary steps include the establishment of an alliance with school supervi-sory personnel predicated on trust and confidence; development of a consultation model that recognizes the intrinsic command and authority structure of the school system; and acknowledgment that mental health expertise and services are always at the service of the school's wishes and dictates, although within reasonable parameters of medical ethics and professional judgment.

The stated task is expeditiously providing services to children; the need to provide consultation, training, and emotional debrief-ing exercises for school principals and teachers, however, is not always recognized. After Hurricane Andrew, my colleagues and I quickly learned that principals and teachers have few identifi-able resources available to them within the school system. More-over, they may decline to avail themselves of these intrinsic mental health resources because of confidentiality concerns.

Nevertheless, DCPS rejected our efforts to develop a group experience for school principals; the regional directors and admin-istrative personnel considered such programs to be their responsi-bility. The school system also resisted efforts to focus on teachers as "silent victims." Such initiatives were always met with the comment that the employment assistance program included mental health support services for teachers. My colleagues and I believe that these services were not well used, however. Although teachers did suffer and continued to suffer throughout the academic year, we had to provide support services informally, outside the school structure.

Yet our efforts with students—that is, the training and assignment of crisis intervention specialists and crisis mobile teams—were quite effective. Crisis intervention specialists spent an average of 65% of their time with children, 15% with parents, 12% with staff/teachers, and 9% on administrative responsibilities. During an average week, the crisis intervention specialists counseled 1,320 individual chil-dren, 880 groups of children, and 352 families; handled 264 crisis intervention situations; and conducted 352 staff interventions.

As I noted earlier, posthurricane psychological distress evolved over the course of the school year. Initially, my colleagues and I found a significant increase in posttraumatic stress symptomatology and a reduction in other indices of psychopathology, including emotional and behavioral problems. Within 3 months after the disaster, disruptive behavior began to rise in the affected area and then gradually abated to levels consistent with the previous year. We attribute this reduction to the effectiveness of the crisis intervention specialists within the school system. One indicator of this effectiveness is the decrease in the reported number of children who attempted suicide in the school year following Hurricane Andrew compared with previous school years: a 20% reduction compared with the previous school year (1991–1992) and a 40% reduction compared with the 1990–1991 school year.

SUMMARY

The school is the social infrastructure within which, through which, and by which effective and comprehensive prevention/intervention services for children can be most expeditiously delivered to the larger community. In the postdisaster period, emotional and behavioral problems—including posttraumatic symptomatology, grief and bereavement, depressive and anxiety conditions, and disruptive behavior disorders—clearly increase; these conditions require a spectrum of therapeutic interventions. My colleagues and I developed school-based programs at the local and systemic levels for the purpose of identifying, triaging, and providing intervention services for the child victims of community disaster.

REFERENCES

Achenbach T, Edelbrock C: Manual for the Child Behavior Checklist and Revised Child Behavior Profile . Burlington, VT, Queen City Printers, 1983

Bloch DA, Silber E, Perry AB: Some factors in the emotional reaction of children to disaster. Am J Psychiatry 113:416–422, 1956

Burke J, Moccia P, Borus J, et al: Emotional distress in fifth-grade children 10 months after a natural disaster. J Am Acad Child Psychiatry 25: 536–541, 1986

Cohen S: Psychosocial models of the role of support in the etiology of physical disease. Health Psychology 7:269–297, 1988

Frederick CJ: Children traumatized by catastrophic situations, in Post-Traumatic Stress Disorders in Children. Edited by Spencer E, Pynoos RS. Washington, DC, American Psychiatric Press, 1985, pp 73–99

Green BL, Korol M, Grace M, et al: Children and disaster: age, gender, and parental effects on PTSD symptoms. J Am Acad Child Adolesc Psychiatry 30:945–951, 1991

Kiser L, Heston J, Hickerson MS, et al: Anticipatory stress in children and adolescents. Am J Psychiatry 150:87–92, 1993

Newman CJ: Children of disaster: clinical observations at Buffalo Creek. Am J Psychiatry 133:306–312, 1976

Pynoos R, Frederick C, Nader K, et al: Life threat and post-traumatic stress in school age children. Arch Gen Psychiatry 44:1057–1063, 1987

Terr LC: Psychic trauma in children: observations following the Chowchilla bus kidnapping. Am J Psychiatry 138:14–19, 1981

Terr LC: Chowchilla revisited: the effects of trauma four years after a school bus kidnapping. Am J Psychiatry 140:1543–1550, 1983

Terr LC: Childhood traumas: an outline and overview. Am J Psychiatry 148:1–20, 1991

Part III

Long-Term Responses to Trauma and Disaster

Chapter 8

Persistence of PTSD in Former Prisoners of War

William F. Page, Ph.D., Brian E. Engdahl, Ph.D., and Raina E. Eberly, Ph.D.

Military combat obviously entails exposure to traumatic events outside the range of usual experience—a prerequisite to a diagnosis of posttraumatic stress disorder (PTSD). Although researchers have studied PTSD among combat veterans most intensively in veterans of the Vietnam conflict, psychiatrists currently regard PTSD as simply the most recent diagnostic term for conditions that physicians in earlier wars called "shell shock," "combat stress," or "war neurosis." Thus, research on PTSD is the latest link in a chain of research in the field of military psychiatry (Kolb 1993).

During World War II, 94,000 American military personnel were taken captive in the European theater; 27,000 were captured in the Pacific theater. During the Korean conflict, 7,000 Americans became military prisoners. Prisoners of war (POWs) in the Pacific theater of World War II and in the Korean conflict were treated very harshly; they generally were starved and frequently were beaten and tortured. The crudest—yet most direct—evidence of the brutality of treatment is the 40% death rate among prisoners of the Japanese during roughly 3 $1/2$ years of captivity.

STUDIES OF A NATIONAL COHORT OF FORMER POWS

In the 1950s the Medical Follow-Up Agency (MFUA) of the National Academy of Sciences assembled and began to study independent samples of World War II Pacific and European theater prisoners and Korean conflict POWs. For roughly 40 years, the long-term follow-up of this cohort, which includes morbidity and mortality statistics collected through military and U.S. Department of Veterans Affairs (VA) records and mail questionnaires, has provided some of the most comprehensive data on the medical and psychological effects of trauma (Beebe 1975; Cohen and Cooper 1955; Engdahl and Page 1991; Engdahl et al. 1991a, 1993; Keehn 1980; Nefzger 1970; Page 1991, 1992; Page et al. 1991).

National Examination Survey

Beginning in 1986, under VA sponsorship, the MFUA began to invite the nearly 2,000 POWs in the sample and an equal number of non-POW veteran controls to undergo a comprehensive medical examination at a nearby VA medical facility. The results of those nearly 1,100 examinations and associated material form the basis for the analysis in this chapter; we report PTSD prevalence data from the latest national survey (Page 1992). Because PTSD is a new diagnostic entity, however, only this latest follow-up (completed in 1992) contained explicit data on PTSD. The latest follow-up also was the first to report results for the entire cohort based on physicians' examinations and structured interviews.

Table 8–1 lists the numbers of subjects invited to take the exam, the number of completed exams, and response rates for each POW and control group. PWP refers to POWs in the Pacific theater and PWE to POWs in the European theater during World War II, and PWK refers to POWs in the Korean conflict; the corresponding control groups are WP, WE, and WK. One additional POW group

Table 8–1. Sample sizes and response rates by study group

	PWP	PWE	PWEM	PWK	WP	WE	WK
Number invited	650	142	222	805	551	302	751
Number of completed examinations	250	36	83	408	54	27	103
Response rate (%)	39	39	37	51	10	9	14

Note. POWs = prisoners of war; PWP = POWs in the Pacific theater; PWE = POWs in the European theater; PWEM = POWs in the European theater who were so severely malnourished that they were hospitalized on liberation; PWK = POWs in the Korean conflict; WP = control subjects in the Pacific theater; WE = control subjects in the European theater; WK = control subjects in the Korean conflict.

consists of POWs in the European theater of World War II who were so severely malnourished that they were hospitalized on their liberation; we refer to this group as PWEM.

Although response rates were low—37%–51% across the POW groups and 9%–14% for control groups—our investigations of response bias found no substantial differences between respondents and nonrespondents. Comparisons of demographic data between veterans who were eligible for the study and those who actually completed an examination found no significant differences in the distributions of year of birth, race, inductee or not, marital status, years of education, or armed service (arms, technical, or Air Force). Also, VA data for the period 1969–1985 (just before the study) showed no statistically significant differences in hospitalization rates between respondents and nonrespondents. These demographic and hospitalization data provide some assurance that response bias is not overwhelming. Furthermore, an earlier investigation of response bias in a 1985 mail questionnaire on depressive symptoms showed a similar lack of substantial bias (Page 1991).

Lifetime PTSD prevalence in the national survey. The 1992 national examination assessed PTSD using three separate measures: a physician's examination; the Structured Clinical Interview for DSM-III-R (SCID; Spitzer and Williams 1986); and a psychological questionnaire, the Mississippi Scale for Combat-Related PTSD (M-PTSD; Keane et al. 1988).

Figure 8–1 shows the lifetime prevalence of PTSD as assessed by the PTSD portion of the SCID. The prevalence of PTSD in most POW groups differed appreciably from the corresponding control subjects, with PTSD rates as high as 31% in PWEM, 33% in PWP, and 41% in PWK. The Korean control subjects deserve special mention for their high rate of PTSD (33%) compared with other control subjects. This high rate probably can be explained by the fact that the WK group, unlike the other control groups, included only men wounded and returned to action. Based on what psychiatrists know about the effects of combat stress, the WK group would be expected to have higher rates of PTSD than the other control groups (although probably less than the POWs).

Physicians' examinations found lifetime rates of PTSD among POWs that were fairly close to the SCID results, as shown in Figure

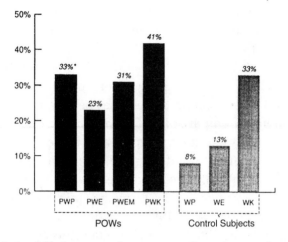

Figure 8–1. Lifetime prevalence rates of posttraumatic stress disorder as ascertained by Structured Clinical Interview. *Statistically significant difference in prisoner of war (POW) and control rates at the $P = .05$ level. PWP = POWs in the Pacific theater; PWE = POWs in the European theater; PWEM = POWs in the European theater who were so severely mal-nourished that they were hospitalized on liberation; PWK = POWs in the Korean conflict; WP = control subjects in the Pacific theater; WE = control subjects in the European theater; WK = control subjects in the Korean conflict.

8–2. Prevalence rates were about 25% among World War II European theater POWs (PWE and PWEM) and about 40% among World War II Pacific theater POWs and Korean conflict POWs. PTSD rates among non-POW veteran control subjects were appreciably lower, ranging from 4% in WP to 12% in WK. By this measure, the WK group has about the same rate of PTSD as the WE group; again, however, WK is an idiosyncratic control group.

Current PTSD prevalence in the national survey. The M-PTSD scale also was administered to examinees as a paper-and-pencil test. The M-PTSD test measures only current PTSD; it yielded estimates of PTSD prevalence among the PWEM and PWK groups that were somewhat higher than those based on the SCID or examining physicians' current diagnoses (all shown in Table 8–2). Further investigations of the differences between SCID, exam, and M-PTSD scale results are in progress.

Lifetime versus current levels of PTSD (SCID). By comparing the data illustrated in Figure 8–1 with those listed in Table 8–2, we

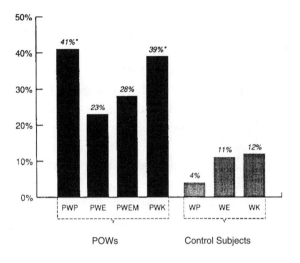

Figure 8–2. Lifetime prevalence rates of posttraumatic stress disorder as ascertained by physician diagnosis. *Statistically significant difference in prisoner of war (POW) and control rates at the *P* = .05 level. PWP = POWs in the Pacific theater; PWE = POWs in the European theater; PWEM = POWs in the European theater who were so severely malnourished that they were hospitalized on liberation; PWK = POWs in the Korean conflict; WP = control subjects in the Pacific theater; WE = control subjects in the European theater; WK = control subjects in the Korean conflict.

Table 8–2. Three measures of current posttraumatic stress disorder rates among former prisoners of war by study group

Study group	SCID	Physician	M-PTSD
PWP	17.3	40.0	32.3
PWE	11.6	20.4	21.6
PWEM	18.8	27.7	38.2
PWK	37.9	37.0	45.4

Note. Rates given are percentages. SCID = Structured Clinical Interview for DSM-III-R; M-PTSD = Mississippi Scale for Combat-Related PTSD; PWP = POWs in the Pacific theater; PWE = POWs in the European theater; PWEM = POWs in the European theater who were so severely malnourished that they were hospitalized on liberation; PWK = POWs in the Korean conflict.

can contrast lifetime and current estimates of PTSD among POWs as ascertained by the SCID. Among the World War II POWs (PWP, PWE, and PWEM), current PTSD rates are roughly half the lifetime rates indicating that roughly half of these POWs who once suffered from PTSD are not currently diagnosed with that condition. The Korean conflict POWs do not follow this pattern; lifetime and current PTSD rates for this group—41.3% and 37.9%, respectively—are nearly the same.

Several hypotheses may help explain the latter finding. First, Korean conflict POWs are younger than their World War II counterparts by about a decade; the prevalence of PTSD may not begin to attenuate until patients reach the current age of World War II POWs—roughly 65–75 years of age. Second, although the PWK group was treated almost as harshly as the PWP group and much more harshly than the PWE group—according to self-reports—its members were not welcomed back and reintegrated into society the way World War II POWs and veterans were. The relatively higher level of current PTSD among the PWK group may be a function of a less satisfactory postcaptivity adjustment. Third, the men who were captured during the Korean conflict differed in various ways from those captured during World War II—on the whole, for example, Korean conflict POWs generally were less well-educated than their World War II counterparts. Other factors do contribute; understanding this unusual finding will require further analysis of examinations and data collected earlier.

Lifetime versus current levels of PTSD (physician diagnoses). The data shown in Figure 8–2 and the data listed in Table 8–2 allow a comparison of lifetime and current PTSD rates based on physician diagnosis. Under this assessment method, lifetime and current rates are very nearly the same—an entirely different picture than that provided by the SCID. This finding may result merely from incomplete recordkeeping, however; because physicians define current PTSD operationally as an unresolved case of PTSD, they simply may not document resolved cases of PTSD. Physicians may respond more to reports of symptoms per se, and they may be less careful in differentiating current from past symptoms. They also may be more likely to diagnose partial PTSD as PTSD, which would be consistent with what we know about diagnoses taken from unstructured interviews. One interpretation, therefore, regards the SCID data as more valid than the usual physicians' diagnoses because the SCID data require more structured note-taking.

Data for other diagnoses. Table 8–3 presents prevalence rates of psychiatric conditions other than PTSD. There are appreciable differences in prevalence rates between POWs and control subjects for depressive disorder as well as generalized anxiety. These differences underscore the most striking major finding of the national examination study—that the psychiatric sequelae of military captivity continue into the fifth decade following repatriation.

Previous studies of this group. The first comprehensive morbidity follow-up of the World War II POW cohort, conducted in 1965–1967 (Beebe 1975), found that psychiatric sequelae were the most striking and persistent aftereffects of captivity. In a 1984–1985 follow-up questionnaire (Engdahl and Page 1991), depressive symptoms 40 years after repatriation—as measured by the Center for Epidemiologic Studies depression scale (CES-D; Radloff 1977)—were three to five times more prevalent in former POWs than in the general population. Furthermore, the rates of depressive symptoms were significantly higher among POWs who reported more medical symptoms in prison camp, had greater weight loss, were younger when captured, or had fewer years of formal education (Page et al. 1991). Similar analyses of the components of the CES-D showed that negative affect, positive affect, somatic symptoms, and interpersonal problems were associated with similar risk factors (Engdahl et al. 1991a). A structural model analysis of depressive symptom data from 1967 and 1985 showed that trauma exposure and individual resilience jointly influenced depressive symptoms (Engdahl et al. 1993). Although depressive symptoms were likely associated with PTSD, such an association could not be directly examined because the 1985 data included no specific data on PTSD.

Summary of National Survey PTSD Results

The SCID data show that roughly one-half of the World War II POWs with lifetime PTSD experienced symptom decline to subclinical

Table 8–3. Prevalence rates of unresolved psychiatric conditions among former prisoners of war by study group

Study group	PWP	PWE	PWEM	PWK	WP	WE	WK
Depressive disorder	46.8	31.7	50.6	51.0	13.0	0.0	22.3
Bipolar I or II disorder	0.8	0.0	0.0	0.3	0.8	0.0	0.0
Alcohol abuse or dependence	12.8	14.1	19.3	27.5	14.8	7.4	32.0
Schizophrenia	1.2	0.0	2.4	3.2	0.0	0.0	1.0
Generalized anxiety	38.8	39.4	55.4	54.2	9.3	7.4	22.3

Note. Rates given are percentages. PWP = POWs in the Pacific theater; PWE = POWs in the European theater; PWEM = POWs in the European theater who were so severely malnourished that they were hospitalized on liberation; PWK = POWs in the Korean conflict; WP = control subjects in the Pacific theater; WE = control subjects in the European theater; WK = control subjects in the Korean conflict.

levels; POWs from the Korean conflict did not show this decrease. Lifetime and current PTSD levels as diagnosed by unstructured interview differ only slightly. Although many POWs apparently have recovered, PTSD rates still are quite high—despite the passage of nearly half a century—not only among POWs but also among non-POW combat veterans. Psychiatrists are only beginning to understand the course of chronic PTSD (Engdahl and Eberly, in press; Solomon 1993).

PTSD PREVALENCE IN OTHER GROUPS

The Epidemiologic Catchment Area study (Helzer et al. 1987) reported a PTSD rate of 0.5% among men in a large sample of the general population; only among a much smaller group of men who happened to have served in Vietnam were PTSD rates appreciably higher. For Vietnam-era veterans who had not been wounded, the PTSD rate was 4%; for wounded Vietnam veterans, the rate was 28%—much closer to the prevalence rates for World War II and Korean POWs, although the follow-up period obviously was much shorter.

PTSD data from a national survey of Vietnam veterans (Kulka et al. 1990) revealed overall PTSD rates of about 15%; the rates among combat veterans were approximately twice as high. Again, these veterans are younger, and the follow-up period is shorter; nevertheless, the PTSD rates are in same range as those reported among World War II and Korean POWs. Compared with the general population, the PTSD rate among POWs is strikingly high by all three measures. Even compared with wounded Vietnam combat veterans, the PWP and PWK groups exhibit appreciably higher PTSD rates.

The results from the national survey also compare with those from other VA studies. Regional studies of POWs by investigators at VA medical centers include results obtained at the Minneapolis VA Medical Center (see Kulka et al. 1990). Investigators examined POWs ($N = 205$) using the SCID and the M-PTSD; the findings paralleled those from the MFUA study. Both studies revealed appreciable variation in PTSD rates by assessment method. With the SCID diagnosis as the criterion, the clinical interview was equivalent to the M-PTSD scale; both exhibited SCID-defined discrepancies across samples in approximately 7%–23% of the cases.

IMPLICATIONS FOR ASSESSMENT

Diagnostic discrepancies may arise because PTSD is an evolving construct that exhibits significant overlap (comorbidity) with other diagnostic constructs (Engdahl et al. 1991b; Mellman et al. 1992). Diagnosis may be further complicated by the differing symptom pictures presented by older trauma survivors because of their age, generational and cohort effects, and time elapsed since trauma (Schnurr 1991). Symptoms may differ in intensity as well as in kind among older trauma survivors.

A study of Dutch World War II resistance veterans (Hovens et al. 1992) identified subjective distress, a confounding factor that may influence a clinician's diagnosis. Diagnostic discrepancies revealed that subjects with PTSD-negative clinical exams and PTSD-positive SCID assessments typically displayed minimal distress levels, leading to a negative clinical diagnosis. The investigators suggested weighting symptom intensity. Certain weighting schemes could decrease PTSD-positive diagnoses among those with lower distress levels, although such approaches would depart from current diagnostic standards.

IMPLICATIONS FOR TREATMENT

Following the foregoing reasoning, a PTSD-negative clinical interview occurring with a PTSD-positive SCID assessment (or moderately elevated M-PTSD score) suggests the presence of chronic, stable PTSD; such a diagnosis, however, may be clinically insignificant, in the sense that focused intervention is not indicated. In other words, patients may report experiencing enough intrusive, avoidant, and hyperarousal symptoms to qualify technically for a PTSD diagnosis but little distress associated with their symptoms. Those expressing little distress may be less appropriate candidates for treatment; moreover, these individuals often decline such recommendations. Such patients are more likely to accept educational and supportive approaches than therapy that is aimed at recalling traumatic memories and treating associated psychiatric symptoms.

Obviously, patients with higher distress levels—as determined via clinical interview—require careful consideration for intervention regardless of their SCID or M-PTSD status. Careful evaluation of possible secondary symptoms, especially depression, is warranted in older trauma survivors regardless of PTSD status.

Sensitivity toward older war veterans is vital. An awareness that their PTSD may have gone unnoticed by other health care professionals for decades should encourage direct clinical inquiries about possible PTSD symptoms. We strongly recommend a structured interview. Although the term "structured interview" may suggest an unnatural process, such an approach need not be (and usually is not) confining; the clinician may introduce the SCID's PTSD module as a "standard" list of questions about reactions people often experience after exposure to trauma.

PTSD symptoms have been all too common, yet underdiagnosed, among older war veterans, especially POWs. Furthermore, the extraordinary persistence and severity of their PTSD symptoms have been baffling and often painful for most of these patients and their families. Psychiatrists should emphasize that they regard PTSD symptoms as expected, predictable reactions to traumatic experiences; war veterans and other trauma survivors often are surprised and relieved to learn that they are not alone in experiencing these symptoms.

REFERENCES

Beebe GW: Follow-up studies of World War II and Korean war prisoners, II: morbidity, disability, and maladjustments. Am J Epidemiol 101: 400–422, 1975

Cohen BM, Cooper MZ: A Follow-up Study of World War II Prisoners of War. Washington, DC, VA Medical Monograph, 1955

Engdahl BE, Eberly RE: The course of chronic PTSD, in Stressful Life Events, 2nd Edition. Edited by Miller TW. New York, International Universities Press (in press)

Engdahl BE, Page WF: Psychological effects of military captivity, in Epidemiology in Military and Veteran Populations. Edited by Page WF. Washington, DC, National Academy Press, 1991, pp 49–66

Engdahl BE, Page WF, Miller TW: Age, education, maltreatment, and social support as predictors of chronic depression in former prisoners of war. Soc Psychiatry Psychiatr Epidemiol 26:63–67, 1991a

Engdahl BE, Speed N, Eberly RE, et al: Comorbidity of psychiatric disorders and personality profiles of American World War II prisoners of war. J Nerv Ment Dis 179:181–187, 1991b

Engdahl BE, Harkness AR, Eberly RE, et al: Structural models of captivity trauma, resilience, and trauma response among former prisoners of war 20 to 40 years after release. Soc Psychiatry Psychiatr Epidemiol 28:109–115, 1993

Helzer JE, Robins LN, McEvoy L: Post-traumatic stress disorder in the general population. N Engl J Med 317:1630–1634, 1987

Hovens JE, Falger PR, Op den Velde W, et al: Occurrence of current posttraumatic stress disorder among Dutch World War II resistance veterans according to the SCID. Journal of Anxiety Disorders 6:147–157, 1992

Keane TM, Cadell JM, Taylor KL: Mississippi scale for combat-related posttraumatic stress disorder: three studies in reliability. J Consult Clin Psychol 56:85–90, 1988

Keehn RJ: Follow-up studies of World War II and Korean conflict prisoners, III: mortality to 1 January 1976. Am J Epidemiol 111:194–211, 1980

Kolb LC: The psychobiology of PTSD: perspectives and reflections on the past, present, and future. J Trauma Stress 6:293–304, 1993

Kulka RA, Schlenger WE, Fairbank JA, et al: Trauma and the Vietnam War Generation. New York, Brunner/Mazel, 1990

Mellman TA, Randolph CA, Brawman-Mintzer O, et al: Phenomenology and course of psychiatric disorders associated with combat-related posttraumatic stress disorder. Am J Psychiatry 149:1569–1574, 1992

Nefzger MD: Follow-up studies of World War II and Korean war prisoners, I: study plan and mortality findings. Am J Epidemiol 91:123–138, 1970

Page WF: Using longitudinal data to estimate nonresponse. Soc Psychiatry Psychiatr Epidemiol 26:127–131, 1991

Page WF: The Health of Former Prisoners of War: Results from the Medical Examination Survey of Former POWs of World War II and the Korean Conflict. Washington, DC, National Academy Press, 1992

Page WF, Engdahl BE, Eberly RE: Prevalence and correlates of depressive symptoms among former prisoners of war. J Nerv Ment Dis 179:670–677, 1991

Radloff LS: The CES-D scale: a self-report depression scale for research in the general population. Applied Psychological Measurement 1:385–401, 1977

Schnurr PP: PTSD and combat-related psychiatric symptoms in older veterans. PTSD Research Quarterly 2:1–6, 1991

Solomon Z: Combat Stress Reaction. New York, Plenum, 1993

Spitzer RL, Williams JB: Structured Clinical Interview for DSM-III-R, Nonpatient Version (modified for Vietnam veterans readjustment study 4/1/87). New York, New York State Psychiatric Institute, Biometrics Research, 1986

Chapter 9

Comorbidity of Substance Abuse and PTSD

**Kenneth J. Hoffman, M.D., M.P.H., and
Jane E. Sasaki, M.D.**

P osttraumatic stress disorder (PTSD) is based on the presence of an extraordinary stressor that evokes psychological and physiological responses in an otherwise healthy human being. The American Psychiatric Association has established criteria to differentiate PTSD from normal bereavement, adjustment disorders, and personality disorders (American Psychiatric Association 1994). Normal bereavement, for example, does not entail the intensity of symptoms that characterizes PTSD. Although adjustment disorders, like PTSD, are associated with identifiable stressors, the reaction is considered maladaptive; in a personality disorder, maladaptive reactions are pervasive even under minimal stress (American Psychiatric Association Task Force 1991).

Although psychiatrists frequently describe substance abuse within the context of personality, affective, and anxiety disorders, they generally do not consider it in the differential diagnosis of PTSD. Nevertheless, comorbidity between substance abuse and PTSD is deservedly becoming an area of increasing research interest (Cottler et al. 1992).

In this chapter, we review the literature and provide a summary of signs and symptoms of basic intoxication and withdrawal syndromes. We also discuss the impact that substance abuse has on PTSD and other common psychiatric disorders, present assessment strategies and treatment approaches, and suggest future research directions.

SUBSTANCE ABUSE AND COMORBIDITY

The relationship between the signs and symptoms of substance abuse and PTSD can cause difficulties in differentiating the two during patient assessment. The first criterion for PTSD involves an extraordinary stressor; substance-abusing patients frequently encounter unusually traumatic stressors within the context of intoxication. The second PTSD criterion involves reexperience of the traumatic event—through dreams, reliving the event, or being in situations that evoke memories of the event. This dysphoric state corresponds closely with the vivid dreams experienced by addicts in drug craving and recovery, often triggered by exposure to the environment in which drug use occurred. The third PTSD criterion, avoidance of the environment and thoughts related to the traumatic event, resembles the denial mechanisms that addicts use to minimize the reality of substance abuse's negative impact. The fourth PTSD criterion—increased arousal, leading to hypervigilance, insomnia, irritability, and decreased concentration—parallels the autonomic arousal symptoms of substance abuse withdrawal. Even the last criterion in the diagnosis of PTSD, duration, echoes the duration criterion for substance abuse diagnoses.

Furthermore, individuals experiencing PTSD may use drugs as a "numbing" tactic. Also, PTSD and alcohol withdrawal may well have common underlying psychobiological mechanisms. Current research implicates limbic structures in the symptoms of alcohol withdrawal and the increased arousal symptoms of PTSD (Charney et al. 1993; Nestler 1993; Schultz 1991; Southwick et al. 1993).

Comorbidity Research

In the early 1980s, researchers addressed the issue of concurrent psychiatric conditions through the Epidemiological Catchment Area (ECA) study. Investigators chose five sites to provide a representative population within each catchment area; they then performed diagnostic interviews for the lifetime prevalence of DSM-III (American Psychiatric Association 1980) psychiatric conditions. For subjects who endorsed lifetime symptoms, the investigators ascertained their presence and severity within the prior 6 months.

Researchers interviewed 2,663 individuals within the St. Louis catchment area. Of these subjects, 430 (16%) had experienced a stressor sufficient to meet the criteria for PTSD; 36 (8%) of the 430 exposed subjects met the criteria for PTSD. Although the investigators did not know the extent of substance abuse among the subjects or whether trauma preceded or followed substance abuse, PTSD was more common among substance abusers (Cottler et al. 1992).

Researchers have conducted few formal studies on the comorbidity of substance abuse and PTSD; those few studies, however, reflect significant intermingling of substance abuse with the manifestations of PTSD. For example, Hyer et al. (1991) studied three groups of veterans in a chemical dependency unit; none of the subjects had a diagnosis of PTSD. The investigators used the Minnesota Multiphasic Personality Inventory (Hathaway and McKinley 1989) PTSD scale (MMPI-PTSD) to establish a PTSD category among veterans who had combat experience and correlated scores on this scale with their alcohol use. The PTSD group had more difficulty with binge drinking than veterans without PTSD.

Blow et al. (1992) evaluated 22,463 alcoholic patients seeking treatment in Veterans Administration facilities during 1 month in 1986. More than 50% of alcoholic outpatients had one or more psychiatric comorbid diagnoses. Rates for PTSD, schizophrenia, and personality disorders were higher in younger alcoholic patients; rates of major depression, anxiety, and organic brain disorders were higher in older alcoholic patients. On Axis V, more than half of the patients with comorbid diagnoses were rated as severely impaired compared with fewer than one-third of alcoholic patients without a comorbid diagnosis.

Page (1992) examined the rates and relative risk of psychiatric diagnoses among World War II and Korean conflict prisoners of war (POWs) and non-POW veterans. The rates of PTSD, depressive disorder, and generalized anxiety were higher in POWs (34.3%–47.6% than in non-POWs (7.1%–16.3%); the rate of alcohol abuse/dependence, however, was slightly lower in POWs versus non-POWs: 20.4% versus 23%, respectively (see Table 9–1). Table 9–2 presents the relative risk of psychiatric disorders in POWs versus non-POWs.

There is clear evidence for genetic factors within the etiological description of alcohol dependence and depressive disorders

Table 9–1. Rates of psychiatric diagnoses among World War II and Korean Conflict prisoners of war and non-prisoners of war veterans

	POW veterans (N = 883)	Non-POW veterans (N = 184)
PTSD	34.3	7.1
Depressive disorder	46.7	16.3
Generalized anxiety	47.6	16.3
Alcohol abuse/dependence	20.4	23.4

Note. Values are given as percentages. POW = prisoners of war; PTSD = posttraumatic stress disorder.
Source. Derived from Page WF: *The Health of Former Prisoners of War: Results From the Medical Examination Survey of Former POWs of World War II and the Korean Conflict.* A Report for the Medical Follow-Up Agency Institute of Medicine. Washington, DC, National Academy Press, 1992, p. 73.

Table 9–2. Relative risk for psychiatric disorders among World War II and Korean Conflict prisoners of war and non-prisoners of war veterans

	Relative risk*	95% cxonfidence interval	
		Lower	Upper
PTSD	4.86	2.85	8.27
Depressive disorder	2.86	2.05	4.00
Generalized anxiety	2.92	2.09	4.08
Alcohol abuse/dependence	0.87	0.65	1.17

Note. POW = prisoners of war; PTSD = posttraumatic stress disorder.
*Relative risk with 95% confidence interval calculated using EpiInfo Version 5.0: Public Domain Software for Epidemiology and Disease Surveillance. Centers for Disease Control, Epidemiology Program Office, Atlanta, GA, April 1990.

(Comings et al. 1991). In a study of 4,042 Vietnam-era veteran monozygotic and dizygotic twin pairs, True et al. (1993) found evidence of significant genetic influences on symptom liability in PTSD. They determined that genetic factors accounted for 13%–30% of the variance in liability for symptoms in the reexperiencing cluster,

30%–34% for symptoms in the avoidance cluster, and 28%–32% for symptoms in the arousal cluster.

Table 9–3 provides a brief description of effects, intoxication, and withdrawal symptoms for commonly abused chemical substances (Ciraulo and Shader 1991). Differentiating more severe signs of intoxication, overdose, and withdrawal from PTSD is relatively easy; distinguishing PTSD from the primary effects and milder signs and symptoms of intoxication and withdrawal, however, may be difficult. Patients may regard the "desired" effect as "self-medication"; this attitude can hinder the practitioner's ability to establish the presence of PTSD as an underlying disorder. Although psychiatrists recognize that patients often self-medicate when they experience depressive, anxiety, or psychotic symptoms, patients with addiction disorders take the "medication" even though their symptoms become worse. Moreover, patients who use such substances cannot be expected to provide a reliable history describing worsening symptoms (Goldsmith 1993).

Researchers have evinced considerable interest about whether substance abuse precedes comorbid psychiatric disorders. In a study of PTSD among substance users in the general population, for example, Cottler et al. (1992) found that sex and drug use predicted the presence of PTSD; women and people who used cocaine or opiates were more likely to have PTSD. In cases in which substance abuse precedes the comorbid disorder, practitioners may regard the substance abuse disorder as primary and therefore consider the substance abuse as the appropriate first focus of treatment. However, substance abuse may follow the manifestations of the first signs and symptoms of PTSD and other Axis I disorders (Anthenelli and Schuckit 1993). In such cases, psychiatrists regard the substance abuse as an attempt at self-medication and focus on treatment of the comorbid Axis I condition.

Regardless of the timing of substance abuse, however, it has an impact on the functional ability of the patient. Practitioners must carefully assess the severity of such functional impairments. Treatment strategies must be based on patient need; because of the heterogeneity of factors leading to a substance abuse diagnosis, identified impairments are far more important than causal factors alone.

Table 9–3. Commonly abused drugs: effects, intoxication, and withdrawal syndromes

Drug	Effects	Intoxication and overdose	Withdrawal
Alcohol	Alcohol is a major disinhibiter that rapidly provides a sense of relaxation. This effect commonly is associated with loss of concentration, poor coordination, increased confusion, drowsiness, clumsiness, decreased appetite, and sleep.	The primary effects of intoxication are enhanced as dose increases. Blackouts, in which an individual is unable to register new memory, are common. At higher alcohol levels, the individual will become stuporous or comatose. Respiration may become shallow and pulse weak. Nausea and vomiting may result in aspiration and respiratory arrest. Almost every organ system is affected.	Early withdrawal begins hours after the last drink, usually with anxiety, insomnia, irritability, agitation, and a startle response. Withdrawal also may include anorexia, elevated vital signs, nausea and vomiting, vivid hallucinations, nystagmus, and seizures. Late withdrawal includes delirium tremens. Nutritional deficiencies associated with alcohol use may lead to Wernicke's encephalopathy and Korsakoff's syndrome.
Nicotine	Like a stimulant, nicotine commonly elevates mood and enhances concentration, producing both arousal and relaxation. The overall effect assists in the stress response; the individual experiences less anger, tension, and depression. Appetite also is suppressed. Nicotine is one of the	Lightheadedness, headache, nausea and vomiting, general weakness, and diaphoresis are the most common symptoms of overdose. Seizures and hypotension, with respiratory arrest, may occur at very high doses.	Irritability, insomnia, poor concentration, depression, stress intolerance, and hunger are common symptoms of withdrawal that can start within hours. Craving for tobacco may occur after years of abstinence.

Opiates	The patient generally becomes euphoric, unmotivated, listless, and fatigued. The pulse may slow; the skin may become flushed with needle marks and abscesses at injection sites. Usually, pupils are constricted and the patient is constipated.	The patient becomes stuporous, with slowed pulse, clammy skin. Nausea and vomiting may occur. Shallow breathing may evolve to pulmonary edema and respiratory arrest.	Autonomic arousal symptoms include runny nose, teary eyes, restlessness, insomnia, excessive yawning, piloerection, abdominal pain, diarrhea, and muscle twitching.
Hallucinogens	The effect of any hallucinogen appears to be highly variable and dependent on the expectations of the user. Some users become euphoric, with an enhanced, pleasurable awareness of their environment; others quietly withdraw. At worst, an individual may become acutely paranoid, with heightened awareness or distorted perceptions of the environment.	Real sensory input is misperceived. The individual may become extremely dangerous—either suicidal or homicidal. Hallucinations of taste, smell, or touch often occur. Frequently, the individual will mix the hallucinogen with other drugs, leading to a potentially wide variety of manifestations.	No specific withdrawal or tolerance syndromes are described. Some hallucinogens, such as LSD, have been reported to cause flashbacks in chronic users years after they stop using the drug.

(continued)

Table 9–3. Commonly abused drugs: effects, intoxication, and withdrawal syndromes (*continued*)

Drug	Effects	Intoxication and overdose	Withdrawal
Cocaine	Less potent but more pleasurable than nicotine, cocaine rapidly produces aeuphoria in which the user becomes highly self-confident, talkative, energetic, and sexually active. The perceived needs for both sleep and food are eliminated. Commonly, the abuser will binge for days, until money runs out. Continued use is reinforced by the fear of a "crash," in which the abuser will become severely depressed. In time, the intense pleasurable effects may be replaced by feelings of paranoia, anxiety, and panic, and the individual may appear highly agitated.	Like the long-term user, the acutely intoxicated person may become highly paranoid, become unable to sleep or eat, lose concentration, and lose all sexual drive. Blood pressure may increase; pupils dilate, and seizure, cardiac arrhythmia, and respiratory arrest may occur. Overdose potential worsens with the fear of withdrawal and craving for more cocaine to avoid withdrawal.	Withdrawal commonly is characterized by either agitated or retarded depression, with extreme sleepiness and irritability, starting within hours and lasting several days. Concentration may be poor, and the individual may become highly irritable, with gastrointinal upset and anhedonia. Craving may be an ongoing problem after years of abstinence.

Source. Ciraulo DA, Shader RI: *Clinical Manual of Chemical Dependence.* Washington, DC, American Psychiatric Press, 1991.

ASSESSMENT OF SUBSTANCE ABUSE

Primary and secondary prevention strategies make initial assessment and treatment simpler and more straightforward than programs without early screening and diagnosis. Canadian psychiatrists, for example, have expressed considerable interest in early assessment and intervention for "at-risk" alcohol users. Screening involves simple CAGE questions and quantity/frequency questions; a positive screen is followed by an assessment using a more diagnostic approach. Advice and assistance are provided as needed. On average, this brief assessment and intervention takes no more than 5 minutes (Anthenelli and Schuckit 1993).

This approach resembles brief assessment and intervention strategies being developed by the National Institute of Alcoholism and Alcohol Abuse (NIAA) and a smoking cessation program developed through the National Cancer Institute (NCI). Studies have shown that brief intervention early within the natural history of addiction is effective (Anthenelli and Schuckit 1993).

Patients with Addiction and Comorbid PTSD

Researchers have designed several instruments with good reliability and validity to assess impairment secondary to addiction. Such assessment may be particularly important in the presence of comorbid PTSD because of the need to track changes and treatment requirements in these complicated cases.

Addiction Severity Index (ASI). The ASI can be used for intake assessment and reassessments. It covers six basic areas: medical status, employment/support status, drug/alcohol use, legal status, family/social status, and psychiatric status. A raw score is obtained for each of these dimensions, and a composite score is calculated. The ASI must be used in an interview setting; it cannot be administered as a patient questionnaire.

The ASI has demonstrated excellent reliability and validity in clinical settings that require assessment of the presence and impact of substance abuse. The ASI is less reliable for young adolescents, among patients with strong antisocial traits, and in patients who are significantly cognitively impaired. Details about specific events are included as comments; in treatment assessment, however, changes in the numeric scoring are highly associated with patient improvement (McLellan et al. 1988).

Clinical Institute Withdrawal Assessment of Alcohol Scale-Revised (CIWA-Ar). The CIWA-Ar is a rapid assessment instrument that allows the health care provider to determine the risk of serious alcohol withdrawal. It takes approximately 2 minutes to administer and has high interrater reliability.

The CIWA-Ar focuses on key physiological and psychiatric symptoms of alcohol withdrawal: nausea/vomiting, tremors, paroxysmal sweats, anxiety, agitation, tactile disturbances, auditory disturbances, visual disturbances, headache, and clouded sensorium. Each dimension is rated on a scale of 0–7 (0 = not present, 7 = extremely severe). Scores higher than 20 indicate a likely need for intensive withdrawal support, although medication may be used for any patient with a score higher than 6. The CIWA-Ar may be repeated as often as necessary until the patient has no need for further medication (Schultz 1991).

American Society of Addiction Medicine (ASAM) Patient Placement Criteria. ASAM criteria provide a framework for a comprehensive biopsychosocial assessment that measures impairment along dimensions similar to the five dimensions described in DSM-III. ASAM criteria place greater emphasis on Axis IV and V issues.

The ASAM criteria assess impairment within six dimensions:

1. Acute intoxication or withdrawal potential
2. Biomedical conditions and complications
3. Emotional/behavioral conditions or complications
   a. Psychiatric (Axis I) conditions
   b. Emotional/behavioral complications of known or unknown etiology (Axis II)
   c. Transient neuropsychiatric complications
4. Treatment acceptance/resistance
5. Relapse potential
6. Recovery environment

Following assessment, the ASAM criteria allow the practitioner to determine the appropriate intensity of medical services: from physician-managed inpatient care to periodic outpatient care (ASAM 1991).

APPROACHES TO TREATMENT

Psychiatric practice within the military offers instructive lessons in the recognition, diagnosis, and treatment of stress and trauma related disorders. Military psychiatrists have led the medical profession in establishing standards in areas of military importance that were of little interest to the civilian sector.

Military physicians recognized the lingering effects of combat—now diagnosed as PTSD—as early as the Civil War; the rigors of World War I highlighted the importance of stress on physical and mental functioning. Immediate, simple restorative treatment provided the best prognosis for return to duty (Glass 1947, 1953, 1954, 1955). DSM-I (American Psychiatric Association 1952) reflected these developments.

The Vietnam experience forced the military to acknowledge the need to assess and treat extensive drug abuse problems (Holloway 1974). This acknowledgment led the military to initiate deterrence drug testing, several worldwide surveys of drug abuse, outpatient treatment programs at every military installation, and the capability to treat drug abuse in an inpatient setting for as much as 6 weeks (Holloway 1974; Holloway and Ursano 1985). The military implemented its drug and alcohol prevention and control program through personnel channels. Although this program requires medical support, it tends to be separate from other medical services. The program focuses on eliminating drug abuse in the workplace. The goal of treatment has been to minimize the functional impairment of the individual; therefore, intervention has not been dependent on diagnosis. If intervention fails, the individual can be separated from the military; separated service members may then receive treatment through the Department of Veterans Affairs or civilian programs.

The mechanism the military chose for its drug and alcohol program suggests a hypothesis about why military physicians initially paid little attention to the comorbidity of drug abuse and PTSD. A traditional psychiatric service operating within this environment has greater interest in Axis I disorders other than substance abuse. Thus, assessment and treatment of non-substance abuse disorders often become segregated from the treatment of alcohol and drug problems.

Treatment becomes especially complex when PTSD and alcoholism are comorbid in an individual who is expected to function within the same type of environment or occupational setting in which the traumatic event occurred, such as after an industrial accident or combat (Machell 1993). For best results with minimal expense, the key to management is early intervention at the subclinical level; primary, secondary, and tertiary prevention are guiding principles.

Primary and Secondary Prevention

Primary and secondary prevention concepts are critical to interventions at the worksite or within the social environment. Primary prevention emphasizes techniques that prepare an individual for uncontrollable risks. Schoolchildren, for example, may develop skills and attitudes that help them to refrain from smoking or using alcohol or other drugs. Similarly, the military would develop plans to minimize the number of casualties. Communities may take action to reduce violent crime and develop enjoyable, drug-free lifestyles. Such actions generally fall outside the scope of medical practice, but practitioners can take an active advisory role within their communities.

Other primary prevention activities, based on taking action before a diagnosis is established, may be more readily available to clinicians. Practitioners may inform "at-risk" alcohol drinkers with PTSD, for example, about the implications of alcohol abuse and advise them to drink less or abstain.

The military has sent rapid-response psychiatric teams and family support personnel to several deployment areas. Debriefing of combat veterans who have been through a battle in which several comrades died might focus on defusing individual attribution of heroism or villainy to the group; expression of the acceptability of soldiers' actions to those they care about is critical. Such intervention can help service members to reprocess events and view themselves as survivors, rather than victims.

Secondary prevention—actions taken after the onset of illness to militate symptoms and shorten the length of the disorder—usually are directed by clinicians. Education programs for primary care providers and screening programs for individuals diagnosed with PTSD can facilitate early diagnosis and treatment of substance abuse in individuals exposed to trauma. Successful early intervention for substance abuse often entails family involvement in treatment plans to alter the support environment.

Tertiary Prevention

Tertiary prevention is directed toward minimizing disability after a clinical diagnosis has been made. Inpatient and outpatient treatment needs should be based on the severity of impairments, as identified in a comprehensive, multidimensional assessment. Hospitalization of a patient—based on the presence of severe intoxication—may be necessary, for the patient's safety alone. In other circumstances, an insightful patient with a drug-free and supportive family and friends and no history of treatment may do well in an outpatient program.

ASAM describes four levels of care: two inpatient levels (medically managed and medically supervised) and two outpatient levels (intensive and routine). Intervention should provide the patient with the least intensive level of care necessary to treat the range of identified impairments; treatment may progress through different levels of care if reassessment indicates that is appropriate (ASAM 1991).

Dual-Diagnosis Units

Relatively few chemically dependent patients have no other significant psychological or medical problems. Dual-diagnosis units have evolved in recognition of the fact that no single template for treatment can manage the complex variety of problems that develop in the context of substance abuse. Regardless of the complexity of problems, however, clinicians must address substance abuse as a primary focus of treatment. Dual-diagnosis units have been established to provide practitioners with flexibility in developing comprehensive treatment plans that maintain the focus of treatment on substance abuse.

Community Support Networks

Twelve-step programs often provide important support systems for alcoholic individuals, substance abusers, and their families/significant others. These programs encourage substance abusers—regardless of other psychological problems—to admit a lack of control over the addictive substance, place faith in a higher spiritual power, review the strengths and weaknesses of prior experience, trust others, reexamine their relationships, make reparations for the injurious effects of their behavior, and help other substance abusers.

CONCLUSIONS

PTSD is a result of traumatic events (including combat) that confront individuals with extraordinarily severe stressors. Psychological "numbing," interspersed with physiological and psychological arousal, characterizes the human response to such stressors. PTSD symptoms may resemble those of depression, anxiety, and other psychiatric disorders, including substance abuse disorders.

Persons with PTSD may use licit and/or illicit drugs as part of an attempt to alter the manifestations of PTSD. A dichotomous approach establishes intervention based on multiple diagnoses, each of which is treated in isolation from other problems. The current trend within the psychiatric profession, however, emphasizes dual diagnosis. Dual-diagnosis (or comorbid) situations demand more comprehensive treatment plans that require expertise across several disciplines.

Ultimately, practitioners must consider the critical role that alcohol and other drugs may play in altering patients' coping responses to external stressors. Any patient who is using a substance that has an untoward effect must discontinue its use. Furthermore, clinicians must advise patients diagnosed with PTSD who are using alcohol or other drugs as a form of self-medication to discontinue these self-defeating efforts. Treatment must focus on initial removal of the drug and support of the patient in a recovery program. In the presence of other comorbid conditions, the intensity of the treatment setting may have to increase; over time, the patient may be expected to return to a less restrictive environment and higher functioning.

Although psychiatrists recognize that substance abuse has been problematic among war veterans, formal studies of alcoholism are rare. Even alcohol use among Vietnam combat veterans has not been extensively investigated. Further research must assess the presence of multiple impairments in need of treatment, determine the optimal treatment planning process, and, ultimately, document treatment approaches that offer the best outcomes.

REFERENCES

American Psychiatric Association Task Force on DSM-IV: DSM-IV Options Book. Work in Progress, 9/1/91. Washington, DC, American Psychiatric Press, 1991

American Psychiatric Association: Diagnostic and Statistical Manual: Mental Disorders. Washington, DC, American Psychiatric Association, 1952

American Psychiatric Association: Diagnostic and Statistical Manual of Mental Disorders, 3rd Edition. Washington, DC, American Psychiatric Association, 1980

American Psychiatric Association: Diagnostic and Statistical Manual of Mental Disorders, 4th Edition. Washington, DC, American Psychiatric Association, 1994

American Society of Addiction Medicine (ASAM): ASAM Patient Placement Criteria for the Treatment of Psychoactive Substance Use Disorders. Washington, DC, American Society of Addiction Medicine, 1991

Anthenelli RM, Schuckit MA: Affective and anxiety disorders and alcohol and drug dependence: diagnosis and treatment. J Addict Dis 12:73–87, 1993

Blow FC, Cook CA, Booth BM, et al: Age-related psychiatric comorbidities and level of functioning in alcoholic veterans seeking outpatient treatment. Hosp Comm Psychiatry 43:990–995, 1992

Charney DS, Deutch AY, Krystal JH, et al: Psychobiologic mechanisms of posttraumatic stress disorder. Arch Gen Psychiatry 50:294–305, 1993

Ciraulo DA, Shader RI: Clinical Manual of Chemical Dependence. Washington, DC, American Psychiatric Press, 1991

Comings DE, Comings BG, Muhleman D, et al: The dopamine D2 receptor locus as a modifying gene in neuropsychiatric disorders. JAMA 266:1793–1800, 1991

Cottler LB, Compton WM III, Mager D, et al: Posttraumatic stress disorder among substance users from the general population. Am J Psychiatry 149:664–670, 1992

Glass AJ: Effectiveness of forward neuropsychiatric treatment. Bulletin of the U.S. Army Medical Department 7:1034–1041, 1947

Glass AJ: Psychiatry in the Korean Campaign, Part I. U.S. Armed Forces Medical Journal 10:1387–1401, 1953

Glass AJ: Psychiatry in the Korean Campaign, Part II. U.S. Armed Forces Medical Journal 11:1563–1583, 1954

Glass AJ: Principles of combat psychiatry. Mil Med 15:27–33, 1955

Goldsmith JR: An integrated psychology for the addictions: beyond the self-medication hypothesis. J Addict Dis 12:139–154, 1993

Hathaway SR, McKinley JC: Minnesota Multiphasic Personality Inventory—2. Minneapolis, University of Minnesota, 1989

Holloway HC: Epidemiology of heroin dependency among soldiers in Vietnam. Mil Med 139:108–113, 1974

Holloway HC, Ursano RJ: Vietnam veterans on active duty: adjustment in a supportive environment, in The Trauma of War: Stress and Recovery in Vietnam Veterans. Edited by Sonnenberg SM, Blank AS Jr, Talbott JA. Washington, DC, American Psychiatric Press, 1995, pp 321–338

Hyer L, Leach P, Boudewyne PA, et al: Hidden PTSD in substance abuse inpatients among Vietnam veterans. J Subst Abuse Treat 8:213–229, 1991

Machell DF: Combat post-traumatic stress disorder, alcoholism, and the police officer. Journal of Alcohol and Drug Education 38:23–32, 1993

McLellan AT, Luborsky L, Cacciola J, et al: Guide to the Addiction Severity Index: Background, Administration, and Field Testing Results. Treatment Research Report, U.S. Department of Health and Human Services (DHHS), Public Health Service, Alcohol, Drug Abuse, and Mental Health Administration, DHHS Publication No. (ADM)88-1419, 1985 (reprinted 1986, 1988)

Nestler EJ: Molecular mechanisms of drug addiction in the mesolimbic dopamine pathway. Seminars in the Neurosciences 5:369–376, 1993

Page WF: The Health of Former Prisoners of War: Results From the Medical Examination Survey of Former POWs of World War II and the Korean Conflict: A Report for the Medical Follow-Up Agency Institute of Medicine. Washington, DC, National Academy Press, 1992

Schultz TK: Alcohol withdrawal syndrome: clinical features, pathophysiology, and treatment, in Comprehensive Handbook of Drug and Alcohol Addiction. Edited by Miller N. New York, Marcel Dekker, 1991, pp 101–115

Southwick SM, Krystal JH, Morgan CA, et al: Abnormal noradrenergic function in posttraumatic stress disorder. Arch Gen Psychiatry 50:266–274, 1993

True WR, Rice J, Eisen SA, et al: A twin study of genetic and environmental contributions to liability for posttraumatic stress symptoms. Arch Gen Psychiatry 50:257–264, 1993

Chapter 10

Posttraumatic Stress Disorder and the Risk of Traumatic Deaths Among Vietnam Veterans

Tim A. Bullman, M.A., and Han K. Kang, Dr.P.H.

Among all postservice causes of death in Vietnam veterans, only deaths resulting from external causes have been consistently more prevalent than in the general population (Anderson et al. 1986; Breslin et al. 1988; Centers for Disease Control 1987; Watanabe et al. 1991). Higher rates of death from external causes—particularly accidental drug overdoses, motor vehicle accidents, and suicides—among Vietnam veterans may be related to a high prevalence of posttraumatic stress disorder (PTSD) among these veterans. Research on the psychosocial and behavioral sequelae of PTSD offers evidence that supports a possible association between these health outcomes.

Diagnosis of PTSD is based on criteria first set forth by the American Psychiatric Association in DSM-III (American Psychiatric Association 1980). One criterion for PTSD is exposure to a traumatic event. Traumatic events related to service in Vietnam that researchers have determined to be risk factors for PTSD include seeing comrades killed or wounded, being fired on, and being wounded (Bullman et al. 1991; Card 1987; Foy et al. 1984; Frye and Stockton 1982). Suicide research also has cited exposure to traumatic events as a correlate of suicides (Beck and Lester 1976; Farberow and Shneidman 1981; Moss and Hamilton 1957).

Numbing or withdrawal from the environment constitutes another criterion for PTSD. This behavior resembles the social isolation and detachment from the external environment—often labeled *anomie*—that researchers have found is associated with suicide (Barraclough et al. 1974; Borg and Stahl 1982; Dorpat and Ripley

1960; Sainsbury 1986). Other behavioral and emotional characteristics, including drug and alcohol abuse and depression, also are associated with both PTSD and suicide (Barraclough et al. 1974; Borg and Stahl 1982; Card 1987; Center for Disease Control 1988). In fact, researchers have cited the occurrence of major depression and suicide as possible outcomes of the chronic phase of PTSD (Scrignar 1984).

Several studies have investigated the extent of comorbidity of other mental disorders, such as drug and alcohol dependency and depression, with PTSD among Vietnam veterans. In one small study ($N = 25$), 84% of combat veterans diagnosed with PTSD met the criteria for at least one additional psychiatric syndrome—including 64% for alcohol-related diagnoses (Sierles et al. 1983). Keane and Wolfe (1990) reported that 70% of PTSD patients had comorbid mental disorders; Roszell et al. (1991) found an even higher rate of comorbidity—94%. Fontana et al. (1992) reported that the comorbidity of psychiatric disorders with PTSD, including suicide gestures, is strongly associated with the degree to which the veteran was personally responsible for death or injury.

Studies have suggested that substance abuse may be associated with PTSD (Card 1987; Center for Disease Control 1988). The increased risk of death in motor vehicle accidents and accidental poisonings among Vietnam veterans may be related to drug and alcohol abuse. In some instances, consumption of alcohol and/or drugs may impair the victim's ability to operate a vehicle. Other deaths recorded as resulting from motor vehicle accidents and accidental drug overdoses might be hidden suicides.

The presence of PTSD as a risk factor for suicide or other traumatic deaths should result in higher mortality rates for these causes among patients with PTSD than among those with no diagnosis of PTSD. Thus, the trauma of exposure to combat in Vietnam may adversely affect not only the psychological health of Vietnam veterans but their physical well-being as well. If there is a significant relationship between PTSD and suicide or other traumatic deaths, early diagnosis and treatment of PTSD becomes even more important.

In this chapter, we report the results of our own study of Vietnam veterans. The primary objective of this study was to determine whether there is a significant association between the presence of PTSD and the risk of traumatic deaths among these veterans.

Specifically, we hypothesized that traumatic deaths such as accidental drug overdoses, motor vehicle accidents, and suicides would be
elevated among patients with PTSD, compared with a similar group
of Vietnam veterans who were not diagnosed with PTSD. We hoped
to determine the extent to which increased mortality as a result of
traumatic deaths is related to coexisting psychiatric disorders.

METHODS

Selection of Study Subjects

We selected subjects for this study after reviewing diagnostic data
for 118,947 veterans within the Department of Veterans Affairs' (VA)
database known as the Agent Orange Registry (AOR). Although the
AOR was established primarily to monitor veterans' complaints and
health problems that might have resulted from exposure to the her-
bicide Agent Orange, any veteran who served in Vietnam is eligible
for inclusion in the registry regardless of exposure to Agent Orange.

A VA environmental physician conducts the initial medical examination and screening of veterans who report for an AOR exam.
Based on the veteran's medical record or self-reported problems,
the physician may then refer the veteran to a VA psychiatrist. The
psychiatrist evaluates the veteran for possible psychiatric problems,
including PTSD.

The psychiatrist determines the diagnosis of PTSD according to
the DSM-III criteria for PTSD. Veterans who received their AOR exam
after 1987 would have been evaluated according to the criteria in
DSM-III-R (American Psychiatric Association 1987), which were
somewhat more restrictive than those in DSM-III.

All of the subjects in this study had received a physical exam,
including psychiatric evaluation for some veterans, between July
1982 and July 1990; the AOR records up to three diagnoses for each
veteran. Personal and service data recorded in the registry and examined in this study include date of birth, race, marital status, branch
of service, and sex. The AOR also includes additional diagnostic data.

The study group (veterans with PTSD) consisted of all 4,247 male
Vietnam veterans on the AOR as of July 1990 who met the criteria
for PTSD described in the International Classification of Diseases,

9th Revision (ICD-9-CM 1989), Code 309.81; we excluded 9 female veterans with a diagnosis of PTSD. For the comparison group, we randomly selected 12,010 veterans from among the 24,043 male veterans with no clinical diagnosis recorded on the registry as of July 1990.

Ascertainment of Vital Status

We tracked the vital status of all study subjects from the date they received their AOR examination until their date of death or August 16, 1990 (whichever was earlier). We terminated follow-up on August 16, 1990, because identification of deaths from various sources after that date was incomplete.

We ascertained vital status by first matching each veteran's social security number and military service number against the VA's Beneficiary Identification and Record Locator Subsystem (BIRLS). This automated system contains records for veterans and their dependents who have received compensation, pension, education, and other benefits—including death benefits for eligible survivors of deceased veterans. According to a study by the National Academy of Sciences (NAS), BIRLS contains the names of at least 94% of all deceased Vietnam-era veterans (NAS 1985).

Of the 16,257 veterans in the study, BIRLS identified 398 as deceased. We requested death certificates for these veterans from the VA regional office or Federal Record Center where each veteran's claim folder was located.

We then matched all veterans in the study against a Social Security Administration (SSA) file of deaths reported through 1990. With this method, we found 12 additional deaths not identified in BIRLS; we requested death certificates for these veterans from the state that the SSA listed as their last place of residence.

We also matched all study subjects against Internal Revenue Service (IRS) files. Although the IRS files did not include vital status, they did list the last state of residence; we used this information to obtain death certificates for some of the deceased veterans for whom we had not been able to retrieve such documentation through locations indicated in BIRLS or SSA records.

After exhausting sources specified in BIRLS, IRS, and SSA files, we still had not obtained death certificates for 197 deceased veterans. We matched these 197 veterans against the National Death Index (NDI). We found 155 of these veterans in the NDI, and we requested death certificates from the state vital statistics offices indicated.

Thus, we identified a total of 410 deceased veterans among the subjects in our study; we obtained 386 death certificates. This total included 123 (92%) of the 134 deaths among veterans with PTSD and 263 (95%) of the 276 deaths among non-PTSD veterans.

Statistical Analysis

We approached the analysis of mortality data in three stages. In Stage 1, we calculated person-years at risk of dying for each veteran from the date of the AOR examination to the date of death or August 16, 1990. Based on these figures for person-years at risk, we made a simple comparison of the relative frequency of overall causes of death, as well as traumatic deaths of a priori interest, between study group veterans and comparison group veterans. We calculated unadjusted rate ratios (RRs) from the crude death rates.

In Stage 2, we used the Cox regression model to account for potential confounders and determine individual and joint effects of a set of variables on the risk of dying from a specific cause (Dixon 1990). This multivariate technique describes the logarithm of the incidence rate for a specific cause of death as a function of the time since entry into the cohort and the number of predictor variables. The model assumes that the effects of each predictor variable are the same during the entire period of observation. Using this model, we obtained adjusted RRs and calculated 95% confidence intervals around the RRs. We also adjusted for covariates, including age at entry to follow-up, race, and year of examination.

In Stage 3, we made an external comparison of mortality rates among veterans to mortality rates among the total male population in the United States based on the standardized mortality ratio (SMR), adjusted for age, race, and calendar year of death (Thomas and Helde 1986). The SMR is the ratio of observed deaths among veterans to the expected number of deaths in the general population. We considered any RR or SMR value to be significantly different from 1.0 when its 95% confidence interval did not include 1.0.

RESULTS

The mean length of follow-up was 4.2 years for veterans with PTSD and 5.2 years for non-PTSD veterans. Veterans diagnosed with PTSD accumulated a total of 17,755 person-years at risk; non-PTSD veterans accumulated 62,680 person-years. The mean age at death was younger for study group veterans than for comparison group veterans: 42 years and 45 years, respectively.

Table 10–1 presents selected characteristics of study subjects. The mean age in 1982—the earliest date of entry to follow-up and the latest date at which all subjects would have been alive—was 31 years for veterans with PTSD and for non-PTSD veterans; 77% of veterans with PTSD and 70% of non-PTSD veterans were white. More veterans with PTSD (33%) than non-PTSD veterans (20%) were divorced or separated at the time of the AOR exam. Slightly more veterans with PTSD (91%) served as ground troops—that is, in either the Army or the Marines—than did non-PTSD veterans (86%); 79% of veterans with PTSD and 83% of non-PTSD veterans had served 1 year in Vietnam.

During the follow-up period, the mortality rate among veterans with PTSD was 71% higher than the rate among non-PTSD veterans. Most of this excess mortality rate was associated with external causes of deaths, such as accidental poisonings, motor vehicle accidents, and suicides. We assessed the possible effects of selected covariates (age, race, year of AOR exam) on the risk of dying from these specific causes by including them in the Cox regression model; adjustment for these covariates did not substantially change RR estimates. As Table 10–2 indicates, PTSD was associated with statistically significant increased risks for all accidental deaths (RR = 2.00), accidental poisonings (RR = 2.89), and suicides (RR = 3.97).

Table 10–3 presents cause-specific mortality for veterans with PTSD and non-PTSD veterans compared with the general male population (adjusted for age, race, and calendar-year period). Veterans with PTSD had excess mortality from all causes (SMR = 2.05). Diseases of the digestive system accounted for one statistically significant elevated cause of death among PTSD veterans (SMR = 2.51);

Table 10–1. Demographic and military characteristics of Vietnam veterans selected for study

Characteristics	Veterans with PTSD (N = 4,247)		Veterans without PTSD (N = 12,010)	
	n	%	n	%
Age at entry to follow-up (years)				
26–36	1,176	28	3,945	33
37–39	1,408	33	4,012	33
≥40	1,663	39	4,053	34
Race				
White	3,285	77	8,427	70
Nonwhite	962	23	3,583	30
Marital status				
Married	2,417	57	8,441	70
Divorced/separated	1,423	34	2,354	20
Never married	386	9	1,094	9
Widowed	21	.5	55	.5
Unknown	0	0	66	.5
Branch of service				
Army	2,864	67	8,383	70
Air Force	142	3	864	7
Navy	243	6	795	7
Marines	995	23	1,943	16
Others	3	<.1	25	.2

Note. PTSD = posttraumatic stress disorder. Percentages may not total 100 because of rounding.

9 of the 12 deaths from digestive diseases among veterans with PTSD were attributed to cirrhosis of the liver (SMR = 2.74).

Furthermore, veterans with PTSD and non-PTSD veterans had statistically significant increased risk of death from all external causes compared with the general population (SMR = 4.25 and SMR = 1.35, respectively). Both groups of veterans also had increased risk for specific external causes. As we had hypothesized, veterans with PTSD were at greater risk for certain external causes than non-PTSD veterans compared with the general population. Veterans with PTSD had an almost sevenfold increased risk for suicide (SMR = 6.74); the

Table 10–2. Cause-specific mortality among veterans with PTSD compared with veterans without PTSD (through August 1990)

Underlying cause of death (ICDA code)	Veterans with PTSD (N = 4,247)		Veterans without PTSD (N = 12,010)		Crude rate ratio	Relative risk[b]	95% confidence interval
	Observed	Crude rate[a]	Observed	Crude rate[a]			
All causes	134	7.55	276	4.4	1.71	1.84	1.50–2.29[c]
All cancers (140–208)	10	0.56	59	0.94	0.60	0.69	0.35–1.36
All diseases of the circulatory system (390–459)	15	0.84	50	0.80	1.05	1.33	0.74–2.41
All diseases of the digestive system (520–579)	12	0.68	21	0.34	2.00	1.95	0.94–4.07
External causes (E800–999)	74	4.17	88	1.40	3.00	2.90	2.10–3.95[c]
All accidents (E800–949)	31	1.75	53	0.84	2.08	2.00	1.28–3.14[c]
Motor vehicle accidents (E810–829)	16	0.90	28	0.45	2.00	1.85	0.99–3.46
Accidental poisoning (E850–869)	7	0.39	8	0.13	3.00	2.89	1.03–8.12[c]
Suicides (E950–959)	26	1.46	22	0.35	4.17	3.97	2.20–7.03[c]
All other causes	23	1.29	58	0.92	1.40		

Note. PTSD = posttraumatic stress disorder; ICDA = International Classification of Diseases, Adopted (9th Revision). [a]Crude death rates per 1,000 person-years. [b]Estimate derived from proportional hazards multivariate model, adjusting for age at entry to follow-up, race, and year of examination. [c]Does not include 1.0.

Table 10-3. Cause-specific mortality among Vietnam veterans compared with all men (through August 1990)

Underlying cause of death (ICDA code)	Veterans with PTSD (N = 4,247)			Veterans without PTSD (N = 12,010)		
	Observed	SMR[a]	95% confidence interval	Observed	SMR[a]	95% confidence interval
All causes	134	2.05	1.72–2.43	276	0.98	0.87–1.11
All cancers (140–208)	10	0.88	0.42–1.62	59	1.11	0.84–1.43
All diseases of the circulatory system (390–459)	15	0.79	0.44–1.31	50	0.57	0.42–0.75[b]
All diseases of the digestive system (520–579)	12	2.51	1.30–4.39[b]	21	1.05	0.65–1.60
Cirrhosis of the liver (571)	9	2.74	1.25–5.21[b]	17	1.26	0.73–2.01
External causes (E800–999)	74	4.25	3.33–5.33[b]	88	1.35	1.08–1.66[b]
All accidents (E800–949)	31	3.40	2.31–4.82[b]	53	1.57	1.17–2.05[b]
Motor vehicle accidents (E810–829)	16	3.51	2.00–5.70[b]	28	1.70	1.13–2.46[b]
Suicides (E950–959)	26	6.74	4.40–9.87[b]	22	1.67	1.05–2.53[b]

Note. PTSD = posttraumatic stress disorder; ICDA = International Classification of Diseases, Adopted (9th Revision). [a]Standardized Mortality Ratio expected on the basis of rates for American men, adjusted for age, race, and calendar period. [b]Does not include 1.0.

increased risk was much smaller among non-PTSD veterans (SMR = 1.67). Compared with the general population, the risk for all accidental deaths and for motor vehicle deaths among veterans with PTSD was twice that for non-PTSD veterans.

Of veterans with PTSD, 1,001 (23.5%) also had diagnoses for additional mental disorders; of these veterans with comorbid mental disorders, 56% were diagnosed with alcohol and drug dependency disorders (ICD-9, Code 303-305), 11% were diagnosed with neurotic disorders (ICD-9, 300), and 10% were diagnosed with depressive disorders (ICD-9, 311). Table 10–4 lists external-cause mortality data for veterans with PTSD and comorbid mental disorders and veterans with PTSD and no comorbid mental disorders (compared with the general population). Although both groups of veterans with PTSD had statistically significant higher rates for each external cause of death, those with concurrent diagnoses had larger excesses of such deaths than those with no additional mental disorders. Veterans with PTSD with comorbid disorders had a nearly 10-fold higher rate of suicide (SMR = 9.81) than the general population; those with no additional comorbid disorders had a nearly sixfold higher rate (SMR = 5.78).

DISCUSSION

Veterans with PTSD had a two- to fourfold increased risk for external causes of death compared with non-PTSD veterans, even after we adjusted for age, race, and year of AOR examination. Furthermore, echoing the results of other studies of Vietnam veterans (Anderson et al. 1986; Breslin et al. 1988; Centers for Disease Control 1987; Watanabe et al. 1991), veterans with and without PTSD had increased mortality rates for deaths from external causes compared with the general population. Among veterans with PTSD, deaths from all digestive diseases and deaths from cirrhosis of the liver also were significantly elevated. Finally, we found that veterans with PTSD who had additional diagnoses for mental disorders had a greater risk of dying from suicide, motor vehicle accidents, and other accidents than those with no comorbid mental disorder.

The presence of PTSD by itself also is an important risk factor for external causes of death, however. Moreover, in this study, we could

Table 10–4. Cause-specific mortality from external causes among Vietnam veterans with PTSD with comorbid disorders compared with Vietnam veterans with PTSD without comorbid disorders (through August 1990)

Underlying cause of death (ICDA code)	Veterans with PTSD with comorbid disorder (N = 54)			Veterans with PTSD without comorbid disorder (N = 93)		
	Observed	SMR[a]	95% confidence interval	Observed	SMR[a]	95% confidence interval
All external causes (E800–999)	26	6.12	3.99–8.96[b]	48	3.64	2.69–4.83[b]
All accidents (E800–949)	14	6.33	3.46–10.62[b]	17	2.64	1.43–3.94[b]
Motor vehicle accidents (E810–829)	5	4.53	1.46–10.56[b]	11	3.18	1.59–5.70[b]
Suicides (E950–959)	9	9.81	4.48–18.63[b]	17	5.78	3.36–9.25[b]

Note. PTSD = posttraumatic stress disorder; ICDA = International Classification of Diseases, Adopted, 9th Revision. [a]Standardized Mortality Ratio expected on the basis of rates for American men, adjusted for age, race, and calendar period. [b]Does not include 1.0.

not determine the importance of PTSD as a risk factor for suicide relative to diagnoses for other mental disorders. Future research might better approach this issue by comparing mortality rates among veterans with PTSD and no additional mental disorder, those with PTSD and additional mental disorders, and those with mental disorders other than PTSD.

This study had the advantage of relying on clinical data rather than self-reported data for the diagnosis of PTSD. Diagnoses of PTSD were made by mental health professionals according to DSM-III criteria.

Nevertheless, this study is subject to several limitations. Because of the selective nature of the AOR, for example, our findings may not be generalizable either to all Vietnam veterans with PTSD or all Vietnam veterans in general. Another limitation concerns the diagnostic data on the AOR: although the diagnosis for PTSD was based on criteria in DSM-III (for some veterans, DSM-III-R), these clinical data were not collected in a structured manner.

Another possible limitation relates to the choice of veterans with no medical/clinical diagnosis as a comparison group. As a result of this choice, we could not determine whether PTSD alone was responsible for the higher rates of external causes of death; a medical illness of any kind—as opposed to PTSD specifically—might provide an alternative explanation for the reported excesses of traumatic deaths. However, studies assessing the risk of suicide associated with an illness as serious as cancer may discount this possibility; these studies reported approximately twofold excesses of suicides among patients diagnosed with cancer (Louhivuori and Hakama 1979; Marshall et al. 1983). The large difference between the twofold excess among cancer patients and our study's sevenfold excess among PTSD veterans would seem to suggest that medical illness is a less important risk factor for suicide.

Our assessment of the importance of comorbid mental disorders as risk factors for specific external causes of death may need further validation. The proportion of Vietnam veterans with PTSD in this study who had concurrent diagnoses for other mental disorders was much smaller than that reported in other studies (Keane and Wolfe 1990; Roszell et al. 1991; Sierles et al. 1983). The AOR may simply underreport concurrent diagnoses for veterans with PTSD, and the increased risk for external causes of death among these veterans may be associated with the presence of comorbid disorders.

We addressed this issue in our study by comparing mortality rates for veterans who had PTSD with comorbid disorders and those with no comorbid disorders with the general population (Table 10–4). Although veterans with comorbid disorders had the greatest risk for each external cause of death, the presence of PTSD by itself was a statistically significant risk factor for each external cause of death as well. Yet the issue of the relative importance of comorbid disorders may ignore the possibility that these comorbid disorders may result from PTSD.

Finally, we were unable to obtain death certificates for 24 deceased veterans. To assess what potential effect the missing death certificates might have had on our findings, we assumed all 13 deceased non-PTSD veterans with no death certificates were suicides and recalculated the relative risk of suicide associated with PTSD. Although the relative risk for suicide associated with PTSD decreased (from RR = 3.97 to RR = 2.62), it was still significantly elevated.

This study's findings of increased risk of suicide and other external causes of death associated with PTSD provide important information for psychiatric professionals concerned with the health of Vietnam veterans. By identifying the group at greatest risk and providing early intervention, health care workers may be able to prevent some deaths among these veterans. Based on reported PTSD prevalence rates among Vietnam veterans of 2%–15% (Centers for Disease Control 1988; Kulka et al. 1990), the number of preventable deaths may be substantial.

CONCLUSION

Vietnam veterans on the AOR had statistically significant increased risks for various external causes of death associated with PTSD. These findings are supported by other research on PTSD and suicides, which suggests a variety of shared psychosocial and behavioral characteristics.

REFERENCES

American Psychiatric Association: Diagnostic and Statistical Manual of Mental Disorders, 3rd Edition. Washington, DC, American Psychiatric Association, 1980

American Psychiatric Association: Diagnostic and Statistical Manual of Mental Disorders, 3rd Edition, Revised. Washington, DC, American Psychiatric Association, 1987

Anderson HA, Hanrahan LP, Jensen M, et al: Wisconsin Vietnam Veteran Mortality: Final Report. Madison, Wisconsin Division of Health, 1986

Barraclough B, Bunch J, Nelson B, et al: A hundred cases of suicide: clinical aspects. Br J Psychiatry 125:355–373, 1974

Beck AT, Lester D: Components of suicidal intent in completed and attempted. J Psychol 92:35–38, 1976

Borg SE, Stahl M: A prospective study of suicides among psychiatric patients. Acta Psychiatr Scand 65:221–232, 1982

Breslin P, Kang HK, Lee Y: Proportionate mortality study of U.S Army and U.S. Marine Corps veterans of the Vietnam War. J Occup Med 30: 412–419, 1988

Bullman TA, Kang HK, Thomas TL: Posttraumatic stress disorder among Vietnam veterans on the Agent Orange Registry: a case-control analysis. Ann Epidemiol 1:506–512, 1991

Card JJ: Epidemiology of PTSD in a national cohort of Vietnam veterans. J Clin Psychol 43:6–17, 1987

Centers for Disease Control (CDC) Vietnam Experience Study: Postservice mortality among Vietnam veterans. JAMA 257:790–795, 1987

Centers for Disease Control (CDC) Vietnam Experience Study: Health status of Vietnam veterans, I: psychosocial characteristics. JAMA 259: 2701–2707, 1988

Dixon WJ (ed): BMDP Statistical Software Manual, Vol 2. Berkeley, University of California, 1990

Dorpat TL, Ripley HS: A study of suicide in the Seattle area. Compr Psychiatry 1:349–359, 1960

Farberow NL, Shneidman ES (eds): Cry for Help. New York, McGraw-Hill, 1981

Fontana A, Rosenheck R, Brett E: War zone traumas and posttraumatic stress disorder symptomatology. J Nerv Ment Dis 180:748–755, 1992

Foy DW, Siprelle RC, Rueger DB, et al: Etiology of posttraumatic stress disorder in Vietnam veterans: analysis of premilitary, military, and combat exposure influences. J Consult Clin Psychol 52:82–84, 1984

Frye JS, Stockton RA: Discriminate analysis of posttraumatic stress disorder among a group of Vietnam veterans. Am J Psychiatry 139:25–56, 1982

ICD-9-CM. International Classification of Diseases, 9th Revision Clinical Modification, 3rd Edition, Vols 1–3. Washington, DC, Med-Index, 1989

Keane T, Wolfe J: Comorbidity in posttraumatic stress disorder: an analysis of community and clinical studies. J Appl Soc Psychol 20:1776–1788, 1990

Kulka RA, Schlenger WE, Fairbank JA, et al: Trauma and the Vietnam War Generation. New York, Brunner/Mazel, 1990

Louhivuori KA, Hakama M: Risk of suicide among cancer patients. Am J Epidemiol 109:59–65, 1979

Marshall JR, Burnett W, Brasure J: On precipitating factors: cancer as a cause of suicide. Suicide Life Threat Behav 13:15–26, 1983

Moss LM, Hamilton DM: Psychotherapy of the suicidal patient, in Clues to Suicide. Edited by Shneidman ES, Farberow NL. New York, McGraw-Hill, 1957, pp 220–241

National Academy of Sciences (NAS): Ascertainment of Mortality in the U.S. Vietnam Veteran Population. Report of Contract V101 (93) P-37. Washington, DC, Commission on the Life Sciences, Medical Follow-Up Agency, 1985

Roszell D, McFall M, Malas K: Frequency of symptoms and concurrent psychiatric disorder in Vietnam veterans with chronic PTSD. Hosp Comm Psychiatry 42:293–296, 1991

Sainsbury P: The epidemiology of suicide, in Suicide. Edited by Johnston R. Baltimore, MD, Williams & Wilkins, 1986, pp 105–119

Scrignar CB: Posttraumatic Stress Disorder. New York, Prager, 1984

Sierles FS, Chen J, McFarland R, et al: Posttraumatic stress disorder and concurrent psychiatric illness: a preliminary report. Am J Psychiatry 140:1177–1179, 1983

Thomas TL, Helde TT: O/E System: Observed Versus Expected Events, User's Guide—Version 3.0. Bethesda, MD, National Cancer Institute, 1986

Watanabe KK, Kang HK, Thomas TL: Mortality among Vietnam veterans: with methodological considerations. J Occup Med 33:780–785, 1991

Chapter 11

Combat Exposure and PTSD Among Homeless Veterans of Three Wars

Robert Rosenheck, M.D., Linda Frisman, Ph.D.,
Alan Fontana, Ph.D., and Catherine Leda, M.S.N., M.P.H.

A necdotal evidence and systematic surveys have revealed large numbers of veterans—especially veterans who served during the Vietnam era (1964–1975)—among the homeless population in the United States (Farr et al. 1986; Gelberg et al. 1988). Surveys conducted during the 1980s indicated that close to half of homeless veterans served during the Vietnam era (Robertson 1987) compared with only 28% of veterans in the general population (U.S. Census Bureau 1989). These data have led researchers to suggest that homelessness might be yet another consequence of military service during the Vietnam War (Robertson 1987)—and, more specifically, of combat-related posttraumatic stress disorder (PTSD).

The National Vietnam Veterans Readjustment Study (NVVRS), an epidemiologic survey conducted in 1986–1987, found that more than a decade after the last American soldier left Vietnam, 15.2% of those who had served in the Vietnam theater continued to exhibit symptoms of PTSD (Kulka et al. 1989, 1990). Among these veterans, PTSD was associated with other readjustment problems, such as substance abuse, troubled interpersonal relationships, and unemployment (Kulka et al. 1990)—problems that researchers also frequently identify as risk factors for homelessness (Rossi 1989). In fact, among Vietnam veterans surveyed in the NVVRS who met the criteria for PTSD, 23.8% reported that they had been homeless for at least a month or more compared with only 8.1% of all Vietnam veterans (Kulka et al. 1990).

The NVVRS and other studies have established that sustained exposure to the fear, rage, horror, guilt, and grief of war can have lifelong effects on mental health and social adjustment. Yet the relationship of wartime military service, combat exposure, and full PTSD to homelessness has yet to receive systematic scientific scrutiny. Researchers have attributed the general increase in homelessness during the 1980s primarily to broad social factors, such as the declining incomes of working people, the shortage of low-income housing, the declining value of public support payments, and the escalating epidemic of urban drug abuse (Burt 1992). Individual factors found to increase the risk of homelessness include unemployment and psychiatric illness, especially schizophrenia and alcoholism (Burt 1992; Rossi 1989). Thus, the association of Vietnam era service and PTSD with homelessness could be a spurious relationship, reflecting the effect of confounding factors associated with both PTSD and homelessness—factors such as poverty, unemployment, substance abuse, and/or psychiatric disorders other than PTSD.

IDENTIFYING RISK FACTORS FOR HOMELESSNESS AMONG VETERANS

Epidemiologists rely on two basic approaches to identify the causes of disease (Kelsey et al. 1986). In the *prospective* or *cohort* approach, investigators observe a sample of individuals, some of whom have been exposed to a hypothesized risk factor over time. If those exposed to the risk factor experience a higher incidence of disease than those who are not exposed, the investigators presume that the risk factor has an etiologic role in the disease. In the *retrospective* or *case-control* approach, investigators compare a sample of people affected by a disease (cases) with an unaffected sample (control subjects) with respect to the presence of the hypothesized risk factor. Under this approach, the investigators conclude that the risk factor has an etiologic role in causing the disease if it is more common among cases than among control subjects (assuming that other factors are equal). The foundation of case-control studies is the fact—demonstrated by Cornfield (1951)—that the *exposure odds ratio* (the odds of exposure to the risk factor among cases relative to the odds of exposure to the risk factor among control subjects) is equivalent to the *disease odds ratio* in a prospective study (the odds of developing the disease among exposed subjects relative to the odds of developing the disease among nonexposed subjects) (Schlesselman 1982).

To assess the relationship of stressors associated with wartime military service (the risk factors) and homelessness (the "disease"), we have conducted a series of studies comparing homeless and nonhomeless samples with respect to veteran status (Leda and Rosenheck 1992, in press), service during a wartime era (Rosenheck et al. 1991, in press), exposure to combat (Rosenheck et al. 1991, 1992), and a diagnosis of PTSD (Rosenheck and Fontana, in press). If wartime military service, combat exposure, or PTSD were risk factors for homelessness, we would expect to find a significantly higher prevalence of these risk factors in homeless samples than in nonhomeless samples.

METHODS

Databases

We derived data on homeless persons for our studies from three data sets. First, we obtained data on the proportion of veterans among homeless persons from previously unpublished data shared by the authors of four methodologically rigorous and frequently cited community surveys of homeless Americans, conducted between 1986 and 1988 (Breakey et al. 1989; Burt and Cohen 1988; Koegel et al. 1989; Rossi et al. 1986).

Second, we obtained more detailed data on sociodemographic status and military service from structured intake evaluations of more than 50,000 homeless veterans assessed in the U.S. Department of Veterans Affairs' national Homeless Chronically Mentally Ill Veterans (HCMI) program (Rosenheck et al. 1989). This program emphasizes community outreach to inform a broad range of homeless veterans about available Veterans Administration (VA) services; it focuses specifically on veterans who experience psychiatric and substance abuse problems. Therefore, data from this sample may be more comparable to data obtained from help-seeking clinical samples than to data from representative community surveys.

Finally, we obtained detailed data on premilitary, military, and postmilitary experiences of formerly homeless veterans who participated in the NVVRS from public-access data tapes (Kulka et al. 1989).

Researchers in case-control studies select control groups that have had similar exposure to factors other than the risk factor under investigation during the period in question (Schlesselman 1982). In our comparison of the proportion of veterans in homeless and nonhomeless samples, we considered veterans of similar age and race, using national data from the March 1987 current population survey (U.S. Department of Commerce 1987), the Census Bureau's annual sample survey of the U.S. population.

We used two control groups in our examination of combat exposure among homeless and nonhomeless veterans. The first control group was a representative national sample of noninstitutionalized veterans from the Third Survey of Veterans (U.S. Census Bureau 1989). To enhance comparability with the homeless sample, we included only veterans in the lowest income quartile from this sample in each military service era. The second control group consisted of veterans in a national survey of VA outpatient mental health clinic users (Buit, personal communication, June 1993; Ronis et al. 1992).

In our examination of PTSD prevalence among homeless and nonhomeless veterans, we compared homeless combat veterans contacted in a VA community outreach program with combat veterans from the same military service eras who received mental health services from VA outpatient clinics. We also compared estimated PTSD prevalence in the homeless sample with PTSD prevalence among Vietnam veterans in the lowest quartile on personal income in the NVVRS.

Analyses

We calculated odds ratios for each of these comparisons reflecting the relative risk of homelessness with regard to veteran status, combat exposure, and PTSD. In our final analysis, we chose veterans surveyed in the NVVRS who had never been homeless as a control group for comparison with those who did report past homelessness; we used structural equation modeling of the sequential influence of various risk factors on homelessness in the comparison of these two groups.

RESULTS

Veteran Status and Wartime Military Service as Risk Factors

In Rosenheck et al. (in press), we combined data from the four community surveys to estimate the proportions of veterans in each of five age cohorts of homeless men and compared those figures with the proportions of veterans in the general population (Table 11–1). The odds ratios indicated that veterans in the post-Vietnam generation (ages 20–34 years) and in the generation between Korea and Vietnam (ages 45–54 years) had a significantly greater risk of homelessness than nonveterans in those age cohorts. In contrast, veterans who served during the Vietnam era (the 35–44 year age cohort) or during the Korean or World War II eras (ages 55–64 and greater than 64) were at no greater risk of homelessness than nonveterans.

Combat Exposure as a Risk Factor

Rosenheck et al. (1991) examined combat exposure in a sample of more than 10,000 homeless veterans evaluated in the HCMI program. We found that 40.5% of homeless veterans who served during the Vietnam era (1964–1975) reported having been fired on during service in a war zone. This proportion was only slightly greater than the proportion of veterans reporting combat exposure in a community sample of Vietnam era veterans (38.4%) (U. S. Census Bureau 1989).

Table 11–2 extends these findings, using previously unpublished data gathered from tens of thousands of additional homeless veterans assessed between 1988–1992 in the same VA program. This table presents data on combat exposure among homeless veterans who served during three wartime eras: the Vietnam conflict (1964–1975), the Korean conflict (1950–1955), and World War II (1941–1946). For comparison, the table displays data on combat exposure among low-income veterans in the national sample surveyed in the Survey of

Table 11–1. Veterans among homeless men (1986–1987) and among men in the general population (1987), by age group

Age group	Data from homeless surveys (N = 2,223)			Current population survey (U.S. estimates, 1987)			Odds ratio for homelessness among veterans	
	Total homeless (n)	Veterans (n)	Veterans (%)	Total (n)	Veterans (n)	Veterans (%)	Odds ratio	95% confidence interval
20–34	939	287	30.6	30,021	3,016	10.0	3.95	3.39–4.58
35–44	576	214	37.2	16,310	6,015	36.9	1.01	0.85–1.21
45–54	412	242	58.7	11,845	5,312	44.8	1.75	1.45–2.15
55–64	251	155	61.8	10,304	7,205	69.9	0.69	0.53–0.91
>64	45	17	37.8	11,550	5,347	46.3	0.71	0.37–1.34
Total	2,223	915	41.2	80,030	26,895	33.6	1.38	1.05–1.85

Table 11–2. Comparison of combat exposure among homeless and nonhomeless veterans, by service era

	All veterans (*n*)	Combat veterans (*n*)	Combat veterans (%)	Odds ratio	95% confidence interval
Veterans in VA homeless programs					
Vietnam era	28,712	11,670	40.6		
Korean era	3,870	1,386	35.8		
World War II era	2,129	1,176	55.2		
1987 survey of veterans[a]					
Vietnam era	490	238	48.6	0.73	0.60–0.87
Korean era	306	124	40.5	0.85	0.66–1.08
World War II era	618	399	64.6	0.68	0.56–0.82
VA outpatient clinics					
Vietnam era	34,855	20,486	58.8	0.48	0.43–0.53
Korean era	9,797	4,683	47.8	0.61	0.56–0.66
World War II era	17,594	12,388	70.4	0.52	0.47–0.57

Note. VA = Veterans Administration.
[a]Includes only veterans whose personal incomes are below the 25th percentile for that service era.

198

POSTTRAUMATIC STRESS DISORDER

Veterans (U. S. Census Bureau 1989), and—because the HCMI program is a clinical convenience sample—in the 1990 survey of VA mental health clinics (Buit, personal communication, June 1993; Ronis et al. 1992).

In each service era, the proportion of combat veterans among homeless veterans was smaller than the proportions of combat veterans in both the low-income general veteran population and the VA mental health clinic population. Five of the six odds ratios were significantly less than 1.0, suggesting that combat veterans were less likely than non-combat veterans to become homeless.

PTSD as a Risk Factor

At the time of intake assessment, HCMI program clinicians document their initial diagnostic impressions, including whether the veteran appeared to experience combat-related PTSD. Table 11–3 presents the diagnosed prevalence of PTSD among homeless combat veterans of each wartime service era. Although these data were based on preliminary clinical assessments, we believe that the prevalence of PTSD among Vietnam combat veterans (45.1%) is valid because it is similar to the prevalence of PTSD (43.2%) estimated in a subset of 627 Vietnam veterans in the HCMI program, which used standardized assessment methods (Rosenheck et al. 1992). Comparison data in Table 11–3 are from the 1990 survey of VA mental health outpatient clinics (Ronis et al. 1992).

The odds ratios reflect the relative risk of homelessness among combat veterans with PTSD, compared with veterans receiving mental health treatment who did not have PTSD. In each case, the prevalence of PTSD among the homeless veterans was lower than in the VA clinic sample. On two of three comparisons, the risk of homelessness associated with PTSD was significantly lower than with other mental illnesses.

Finally, we compared the proportion of homeless Vietnam veterans diagnosed with PTSD in the HCMI program with the proportion of low-income Vietnam veterans in the NVVRS community sample who met the criteria for PTSD, using the 89-community sample cutoff score on the Mississippi Scale for Combat-Related PTSD (Keane et al. 1988). The resulting PTSD prevalence estimates

Table 11–3. Diagnosed PTSD among homeless combat veterans and combat veterans in VA mental health outpatient clinics, by service era

	Veterans in VA homeless programs			VA outpatient clinics			Odds ratio	95% confidence interval
	All veterans (*n*)	PTSD (*n*)	PTSD (%)	All veterans (*n*)	PTSD (*n*)	PTSD (%)		
Vietnam era	11,670	5,267	45.1	20,486	9,446	46.1	0.96	0.82–1.11
Korean era	1,386	163	11.8	4,683	663	14.2	0.81	0.67–0.97
World War II era	1,176	89	7.6	12,388	2,079	16.8	0.41	0.32–0.51

Note. PTSD = posttraumatic stress disorder. VA = Veterans Administration.

(42.9% in the HCMI sample versus 46.4% in the low-income NVVRS sample) did not yield a significant risk ratio for homelessness resulting from PTSD (odds ratio = 0.87, 95% confidence interval = 0.68–1.07).

Structural Equation Modeling of Past Homelessness

The third source of information on the antecedents of homelessness among veterans was the rich data set available from the NVVRS. Rosenheck and Fontana (in press) carefully reanalyzed these data, using structural equation modeling techniques, to investigate the contribution of numerous health status and social adjustment factors to past homelessness. Among the factors examined were premilitary personal experiences, exposure to war zone stress (including a continuous measure of combat exposure), current PTSD, other psychiatric disorders, and substance abuse.

The most important clinical risk factors for homelessness in these analyses were alcohol and psychiatric illnesses other than PTSD. PTSD had no statistically significant relationship to homelessness independent of other factors. Military service variables had a modest total relationship with past homelessness, with a significant contribution coming from high levels of combat exposure and from participation in atrocities.

DISCUSSION

Before discussing these results, we must acknowledge several limitations of these studies. First, although the sampling strategies used in the community surveys were carefully designed and implemented, data on military service in those surveys were limited to simple determinations of service in the armed forces. Second, although more detailed data on military service and the prevalence of PTSD were available from intake assessments from the VA's homeless program and from the survey of VA mental health clinics, the combat indicator did not reflect the degree of combat exposure. Furthermore, diagnostic data were based on clinical assessments rather than standardized test scores, and both sources of data were convenience samples rather than population-based probability samples. Finally, the NVVRS, although rich in standardized clinical data and based on a national sampling framework, included only rudimentary information on past homelessness. Thus, although the results of these studies were generally consistent with one another, they should be regarded as suggestive rather than conclusive.

Review of Findings

In none of the studies did wartime service, combat exposure, or PTSD appear to be more frequent among currently homeless veterans than among comparison subjects. In the NVVRS sample, however, veterans who were exposed to higher levels of combat stress and veterans who participated in atrocities were more likely to report past homelessness. With this exception, the data offer little support for the expected causal relationship between homelessness and wartime military service, combat exposure, or PTSD. In fact, the only two groups of veterans who appeared to be at greater than expected risk for current homelessness were those who served in peacetime. The higher risk of homelessness among these veterans may reflect the fact that peacetime military personnel policies allow less well-adjusted recruits to join the armed forces in the first place (Janowitz 1975; Laurence et al. 1989; Rosenheck et al. in press).

Veterans Among the Homeless Population

Our findings provide a reminder that, in spite of abundant evidence that wartime trauma can result in prolonged PTSD and other problems, veterans—including veterans of war-zone service—are, in many respects, as well off (or better off) than other Americans. Annual reports from the VA during the 1980s consistently indicated that the median income of male veterans was higher than the median income of age and gender-matched nonveterans (Veterans Administration 1988), and the NVVRS showed that veterans who served in the Vietnam theater had higher incomes than those who served during the Vietnam era but did not serve in Vietnam (Kulka et al. 1990). In addition, the VA, state veterans assistance offices, and veteran service organizations offer veterans a broad array of financial, educational, and health care services that are not available to nonveterans.

The growth of homelessness in this country since 1980 is a symptom of far reaching changes in the American economy and in American society (Danziger and Gottschalk 1993). The three decades after World War II were a period of unprecedented economic growth, during which homelessness was less common than at any previous time in American history (Rossi 1989). During the recession of the early 1980s, however (when unemployment briefly reached Depression-era levels), homeless people became increasingly visible on city streets across the country—an apparent consequence of the recession. Homelessness continued to increase during the following years, despite renewed economic expansion and high employment (U.S. Conference of Mayors 1987). By the end of the 1980s, economists recognized that the years from 1979 to 1989 had seen a dramatic redistribution of wealth in the United States: while incomes increased by 17% among the richest fifth of the population, they declined by 7.6% among the poorest fifth of families (Mishel and Frankel 1991).

This redistribution of income—itself a consequence of changes in the world economy that have put low-income American workers at a serious disadvantage in world labor markets (Reich 1991)—may be the best explanation for the overall growth of homelessness. Thus, although PTSD affects a small but substantial segment of the veteran population (about 470,000 of 8.2 million Vietnam-era veterans), homelessness and the forces that produce it have had a far more widespread impact; they have affected veterans as they have affected many other segments of our society. The story of homeless veterans is a story of America much more than it is a story of Vietnam.

One of the distinctive features of democratic society in the United States is that military service, at all levels, is the responsibility and obligation of the citizenry, not an aristocratic elite. Although some researchers have claimed that the armed forces—especially during the Vietnam war—have drawn disproportionately from lower socioeconomic classes (Appy 1993), the preponderance of studies show that American military forces have been generally representative of the male population (Berryman 1988). Thus, the presence of large numbers of veterans, especially Vietnam-era veterans, among the homeless population may be attributable to three factors: 1) there are large numbers of veterans among the male citizens of the United States; 2) the age range at which men are most vulnerable for homelessness (35–45 years) (Rossi 1989) is the age range of the Vietnam-era veteran population; and 3) veterans are subject to the same social and economic currents as other Americans. In other words, there are so many veterans among the homeless population precisely because the United States has a representative, citizen-based military, rather than one based on a societal elite.

Clinical Implications

Our analysis indicates that wartime military service is not a major independent cause of homelessness. Given this finding, how should practitioners consider past military service and PTSD in the treatment of homeless veterans?

First, even if military service is not a major cause of homelessness among veterans, more than two-fifths of our clinical sample of homeless combat veterans did exhibit war-related PTSD. These veterans unquestionably are entitled to treatment and compensation to the extent that they have illnesses related to their military service.

Second, veteran status—especially wartime service—may play an important role in treatment and rehabilitation. Demoralization and self-doubt are barriers that virtually all homeless persons must overcome as they attempt to reenter mainstream society. Many veterans recall their military service with great pride—as a time when they endured and overcame great hardship. Clinical programs that tap and enlarge this reservoir of pride may rekindle a self-respect that can enhance participation in treatment and increase the likelihood of exiting from homelessness (Rosenheck et al. 1992; Smith and Yates 1992).

Policy Implications

Finally, we must consider the implications of our analysis for public policy toward homeless veterans. Citing a finding that military service does not directly contribute to homelessness, some observers may claim that homelessness among veterans is a local issue and that the federal government need not make special efforts to provide assistance. Two lines of reasoning argue against this position—the first based on the American tradition of collective responsibility for indigent veterans, the second on our national commitment to human rights.

Since the time of Plymouth Colony, Americans have endorsed and conscientiously upheld the nation's responsibility to assist veterans injured in the course of military service (Adkins 1968), although public attitudes toward veterans with impairments not specifically incurred in combat or other service-related duties have been mixed. On one hand, some Americans have been strong veterans' advocates: Corporal J. M. Tanner (Secretary of the Treasury in the 1880s), for example, said he would "drive a six-mule team through the treasury" for Union veterans of the Civil War; once in office, he proceeded to do so (Skocpol 1992). On the other hand, leaders such as Alexander Hamilton and Franklin Roosevelt—although unquestioned patriots—have argued that pensions and other benefits for nonservice-connected veterans place an unwarranted burden on the federal treasury (Ross 1969; Severo and Milford 1989).

Since the end of World War II, the VA health care system has grown to 172 facilities; these facilities provide health care services to millions of indigent nonservice-connected veterans each year. In addition, the federal government provides $2.4 billion annually to more than 600,000 wartime veterans in the form of nonservice-connected pension payments (Veterans Administration 1988). Notably, however, in 1946 the Veterans Emergency Housing Program—a program that would have provided low-income housing to poorer veterans—failed to garner enough support to become law (Ross 1969). With that decision, the broad scope of veterans benefits stopped short of providing low-income veterans with the type of housing subsidies that would be particularly helpful to homeless veterans now.

Nevertheless, many Americans feel that veterans who served the nation in wartime should not be left to fend for themselves when faced with homelessness, even if they have no specific statutory claim to special assistance. Government leaders recognize this responsibility to provide rehabilitative opportunities for veterans, as VA and congressional support for nearly 100 specialized outreach, treatment, and rehabilitation programs for homeless veterans that have been established during the past 7 years—at a time of severe budgetary constraint—demonstrates.

Even in the absence of an explicit legislative mandate to assist homeless veterans, the government's endorsement of the Universal

Declaration of Human Rights (passed by the United Nations General Assembly on December 10, 1948) reiterates the nation's commitment to attend to the needs of all homeless persons. Section 25 of that Declaration asserts that "Everyone has the right to a standard of living adequate to the health and well-being of himself and of his family, including food, clothing, housing and medical care and necessary social services. . . ." Although no nation, sadly, has achieved full compliance with this section—or many of the other 29 articles of the Universal Declaration of Human Rights—many Americans agree that citizens who serve and sacrifice for the nation in time of war clearly deserve these most fundamental of entitlements.

REFERENCES

Adkins R: Medical Care for Veterans. Washington, DC, U.S. Government Printing Office, 1968

Appy C: Working-Class War: American Combat Soldiers and Vietnam. Chapel Hill, University of North Carolina Press, 1993

Berryman SE: Who Serves? The Persistent Myth of the Underclass Army. Boulder, CO, Westview Press, 1988

Breakey W, Fisher P, Kramer M, et al: Health and mental health problems of homeless men and women in Baltimore. JAMA 262:1352–1361, 1989

Burt M: Over the Edge: The Growth of Homelessness in the 1980s. New York, Russell Sage Foundation and Urban Institute Press, 1992

Burt M, Cohen BE: Feeding the Homeless: Does the Prepared Meals Provision Help? Washington, DC, Urban Institute, 1988

Cornfield J: A method of estimating comparative rates from clinical data: applications to cancer of the lung, breast and cervix. J Natl Cancer Inst 11:1269–1275, 1951

Danziger S, Gottschalk P: Uneven Tides: Rising Inequality in America. New York, Russell Sage Foundation, 1993

Farr RK, Koegel P, Burnam A: A Study of Homeless and Mentally Ill in the Skid Row Area of Los Angeles. Los Angeles, CA, Los Angeles County Department of Mental Health, 1986

Gelberg L, Linn LS, Leake L: Mental health, alcohol and drug use and criminal history among homeless adults. Am J Psychiatry 145:191–196, 1988

Janowitz M: The all-volunteer military as a socio-political problem. Social Problems 22:432–449, 1975

Keane TM, Caddell JM, Taylor KL: Mississippi Scale for Combat-Related Posttraumatic Stress Disorder: three studies. J Consult Clin Psychol 56:1–6, 1988

Kelsey JL, Thompson WD, Evans AS: Observational Epidemiological Studies. Oxford, England, Oxford University Press, 1986

Koegel P, Burnam A, Farr R: The prevalence of specific psychiatric disorders among homeless individuals in the inner-city of Los Angeles. Arch Gen Psychiatry 45:1085–1092, 1989

Kulka RA, Schlenger WE, Fairbank JA, et al: Trauma and the Vietnam War Generation: Report of Findings from the National Vietnam Veterans Readjustment Study. New York, Brunner/Mazel, 1989

Kulka RA, Schlenger WE, Fairbank JA, et al: The National Vietnam Veterans Readjustment Study: Tables of Findings and Technical Appendices. New York, Brunner/Mazel, 1990

Laurence JH, Ramsberger PF, Gribben MA: Effects of Military Experience on the Post-Service Lives of Low-Aptitude Recruits: Project 100,000 and the ASVAB Misnorming. Alexandria, VA, Human Resources Research Organization, 1989

Leda CL, Rosenheck RA: Mental illness in homeless female veterans. Hosp Community Psychiatry 43:1026–1028, 1992

Mishel L, Frankel DM: The State of Working America. Armonk, NY, Sharpe, 1991

Reich R: The Work of Nations. New York, Vintage, 1991

Robertson M: Homeless veterans: an emerging problem? in The Homeless in Contemporary Society. Edited by Bingham RD, Green RE, White SB. Beverly Hills, CA, Sage, 1987, pp 201–215

Ronis D, Bates EW, Wolff N: 1990 Survey of Outpatient Mental Health and Readjustment Counseling Services: Analyses of Diagnoses and Problems. Ann Arbor, MI, Great Lakes Health Services Research and Development Field Program, 1992

Rosenheck RA, Fontana A: A model of homelessness among male veterans of the Vietnam generation. Am J Psychiatry (in press)

Rosenheck R, Leda C, Gallup P, et al: Initial assessment data from a 43-site program for homeless chronically mentally ill veterans. Hosp Community Psychiatry 40:937–942, 1989

Rosenheck RA, Gallup P, Leda CL: Vietnam era and Vietnam combat veterans among the homeless. Am J Public Health 81:643–664, 1991

Rosenheck RA, Leda C, Gallup PG: Combat stress, psycho-social adjustment and health services utilization among homeless Vietnam theater veterans. Hosp Community Psychiatry 43:145–149, 1992

Rosenheck RA, Frisman LK, Chung A: The proportion of veterans among the homeless. Am J Public Health (in press)

Ross DRB: Preparing for Ulysses: Politics and Veterans During World War II. New York, Columbia University Press, 1969

Rossi P: Down and Out in America: The Causes of Homelessness. Chicago, IL, University of Chicago Press, 1989

Rossi PH, Fisher GA, Willis G: The Condition of the Homeless in Chicago. Amherst, MA, Social and Demographic Research Institute, 1986

Schlesselman JJ: Case-Control Studies: Design, Conduct, Analysis. Oxford, England, Oxford University Press, 1982

Severo R, Milford L: The Wages of War. New York, Touchstone, 1989

Skocpol T: Protecting Soldiers and Mothers: The Political Origins of Social Policy in the United States. Cambridge, MA, Harvard University Press, 1992

Smith K, Yates J: The New England shelter for homeless veterans: a unique approach. New England Journal of Public Policy 8:669–684, 1992

U.S. Census Bureau: 1987 Survey of Veterans. Washington, DC, Department of Veterans Affairs, 1989

U.S. Conference of Mayors: Status Report on Homeless Families in America's Cities: A 29-City Survey. Washington, DC, U.S. Conference of Mayors, 1987

U.S. Department of Commerce, Bureau of the Census: Current Population Survey: Annual Demographic File, Ann Arbor MI, Inter-University Consortium for Political and Social Research, 1987

Veterans Administration: Annual Report 1987. Washington, DC, Veterans Administration, 1988

Chapter 12

Acute to Chronic: Etiology and Pathophysiology of PTSD—A Biopsychological Approach

Arieh Y. Shalev, M.D.

T he mental sequelae of severe trauma have received various names, including nostalgia, soldier's heart, railway spine, "shell shock," combat neurosis, and combat fatigue. Each of these names reflects a specific conceptual framework such as neuroses, psycho-organic impacts, or existential ailments.

The definition of posttraumatic stress disorder (PTSD) in DSM-III (American Psychiatric Association 1980) and DSM-III-R (American Psychiatric Association 1987) refers to Cannon's (1932) and Selye's (1956) homeostatic model of stress response and "general adaptation syndrome." PTSD is an exception within that model, however. It is an unremitting, self-perpetuating condition for which equilibrium and homeostasis seem to have lost their role of organizing attractors. Furthermore, the central features of this stress syndrome (i.e., reexperiencing and avoidance) reflect a sequence of psycho-analytical observations that includes Freud's (1917/1957) work on grief and mourning, Lindemann's (1944) traumatic loss, and Horowitz's (1974) stress response syndrome.

Effective approaches to the treatment of this syndrome derive from the behavioral model of learned conditioning (e.g., Foa and Rothbaum 1989; Keane et al. 1985). Some of the finest formulations of PTSD are neurobiological (e.g., Charney et al. 1993; Kolb 1987; van der Kolk et al. 1985).

In this chapter, I outline the main explanatory models of PTSD and their clinical implications; this critical review of psychophysiological studies illustrates a unifying approach to complex experimental data. I argue that a multidimensional, biopsychosocial model best accounts for the mental sequelae of severe psychological trauma, and I contend that many of the neurobiological scars left by massive psychological trauma are indelible and require a rehabilitative rather than a curative approach.

BIOLOGICAL MODELS OF PTSD

Research into the psychobiology of PTSD has followed two paths. The first path consists of a search for commonalities between biological mechanisms in PTSD and those of other mental disorders. The second consists of a quest for specific attributes of PTSD.

Similarities Between PTSD and Other Mental Disorders

Comorbid panic disorder appears in 13%–19% of PTSD patients (Bleich et al. 1986; McFarlane 1992; Mellman et al. 1992). Symptoms of phasic arousal in PTSD (e.g., flashbacks, intrusive recollection) resemble panic attacks, and experimental procedures that elicit panic attacks in panic disorder patients, such as yohimbine or lactate infusion (Morgan et al. 1990), can elicit anxiety, dissociation, and flashbacks in PTSD patients. Theoretical formulations based on these findings assign a role to the locus ceruleus-norepinephrine (LC-NE) "alarm" system in PTSD and predict that antipanic medication and clonidine would have a positive effect on PTSD symptoms.

Major depression is frequently codiagnosed in PTSD patients (Davidson et al. 1990; Engdahl et al. 1991; Roszell et al. 1991; Sierles et al. 1983). Depressive symptoms resemble DSM-III-R PTSD symptoms of "diminished interest," "restricted range of affect," and "sense of foreshortened future." Dysregulation of peripheral $\alpha2$ receptors and related second messengers provides preliminary support for the PTSD-depression relationship; treatment modalities based on that relationship involve antidepressants and monoamine oxidase (MAO) inhibitors.

Researchers have interpreted reports of comorbid obsessive-compulsive disorder (OCD) in PTSD (e.g., Pitman 1993) and similarities between the repeated "rumination" of traumatic memories and obsessions as suggesting a common neurobiological mechanism. Specific serotonin reuptake inhibitors (SSRIs) are especially effective in OCD; I review studies of such drugs here.

Specific Biological Attributes of PTSD

Specific models of PTSD entail dysregulation of opioid neuro-modulation, imprinting and consolidation of traumatic memories, and hypothalamic-pituitary-adrenal (HPA) axis dysregulation.

The opioid model (e.g., van der Kolk et al. 1985) suggests that the spontaneous repetition of distressful memories, the presence of self-inflicted injuries, and the repeated self-exposure that typifies trauma survivors results from an "addiction to trauma," mediated by a dysfunctional brain opioid system. A study showing that naloxone, an opiate antagonist, reverses stress-induced analgesia in PTSD (Pitman et al. 1990) partially supports this hypothesis.

The memory imprinting model implies that the "etching" of traumatic experiences into a patient's neuronal network plays a major role in the etiology of the disorder. Stress hormones that are present during the traumatic event may mediate the consolidation of traumatic memories (Pitman 1989). Subsequent development of this model has suggested that traumatic memories are stored "forever" at subcortical levels (e.g., Shalev et al. 1992c), thereby explaining problems in their extinction over time.

The kindling model of PTSD (e.g., Krystal et al. 1989) is a variation of the memory imprinting paradigm; according to this model, repeated processing of distressful recollections lowers the threshold for neuronal transmission of similar signals, thereby "biasing" the brain toward fear and arousal. Importantly, this model extends the time interval during which "traumatic imprinting" takes place into the postexposure period. It implies that intense arousal during a critical period after the trauma is pathogenic. Accordingly, psychiatrists believe that interventions aimed at reducing hyperarousal among recent trauma survivors (e.g., early use of tranquilizers, withdrawal from sources of stress, interpersonal interventions) have the potential to prevent PTSD. This model also predicts an association between secondary stressors (those that follow the impact phase of traumatic events) and long-term psychopathology.

Studies of the HPA "stress" axis (e.g., Mason et al. 1990) have found decreased epinephrine/cortisol ratios, elevated urinary catecholamines, and increased dexamethasone suppression (Yehuda et al. 1993). Findings of cortisol "hypersuppression" in PTSD contrast with findings of blunted response to dexamethasone in depression, suggesting differences in the neurophysiology of the two conditions.

Biological Treatment of PTSD

Pharmacotherapy in PTSD includes all families of psychotropic drugs. Investigators have conducted some major studies (e.g., Davidson 1992; Friedman 1988; S. D. Solomon et al. 1992) (Table 12–1). Studies of antidepressants suggest that these drugs significantly affect core PTSD symptoms and associated depression, insomnia, and anxiety. The magnitude of the response, however, is less than that in patients with major depression or panic disorder. Moreover, three placebo-controlled, double-blind studies (Davidson et al. 1993; Reist et al. 1989; Shestatzky et al. 1988) and one open trial (Lerer et al. 1987) failed to show major effects by antidepressants on core PTSD symptoms. Trials of fluoxetine (Nagy et al. 1993; Shay 1991; van der Kolk et al., 1994) suggest that this SSRI specifically affects core PTSD symptoms. Other studies suggest that lithium (Irwin et al. 1989) and clonidine (Kinzie and Leung 1989) may enhance the effect of antidepressants on PTSD.

Studies of benzodiazepines have produced mixed results. One controlled study (Braun et al. 1990) failed to show a specific effect of alprazolam on PTSD symptoms, despite a modest effect on anxiety. An open study of clonazepam (Loewenstein et al. 1988) described improved sleep and reduction in nightmares, flashbacks, and panic attacks. Risse et al. (1990) described severe withdrawal symptoms, however, in PTSD patients treated with alprazolam.

The results of open trials of mood stabilizers such as lithium, sodium valproate, and carbamazepine suggest that these drugs reduce irritability and improve impulse control in PTSD (e.g., Lipper et al. 1986). In addition, researchers have postulated that the "antikindling" effect of carbamazepine and sodium valproate may hold particular promise for the treatment of PTSD; investigators have not empirically confirmed this claim, however.

Psychopharmacological studies of PTSD display numerous shortcomings (S. D. Solomon et al. 1992). Investigators have conducted few controlled studies, and the results have been inconsistent. Also, most of this research has focused on male combat veterans with chronic PTSD. Although theoretical considerations suggest that early treatment may help to prevent PTSD, researchers have not studied the effect of early pharmacological intervention. Some reviewers (Davidson 1992; Friedman 1988; S. D. Solomon et al. 1992) believe

Table 12–1. Pharmacological treatment of PTSD

Author(s)	Drug	Design	Population	N	Results/conclusions
Antidepressants					
Bleich et al. (1986)	Amitriptyline	OT	Veterans	14	Improved sleep, memory, and concentration; decreased nightmares
	Doxepin Maprotiline Clomipramine			7 2 2	
Davidson et al. (1990)	Amitriptyline Placebo	DB, PC	Miscellaneous PTSD	40	Significant effect on depression and anxiety, modest effect on PTSD Sx
Davidson et al. (1993)	Amitriptyline	DB, PC	War veterans	55	Significant effect on depression & severity index, trend in PTSD Sx
Irwin et al. (1989)	Antidepressants and lithium	CR	Veterans, PTSD,	8	Five of eight cases improved and depression
Kinzie and Leung (1989)	Clonidine and imipramine	OT	Refugees	9	Reduction in depression, nightmares, hyperarousal intrusion Sx
Kosten et al. (1991)	Phenelzine Imipramine	RA, PC	Veterans	19 23	Phenelzine > imipramine > placebo. Reduction in

(continued)

Table 12–1. Pharmacological treatment of PTSD (*continued*)

Author(s)	Drug	Design	Population	N	Results/conclusions
	Placebo			18	intrusive Sx unrelated to antidepressant effect
Nagy et al. (1993)	Fluoxetine	OT	Veterans	27	Reduction in PTSD Sx, unrelated to comorbid panic
Reist et al. (1989)	Desipramine Placebo	DB, PC, CO	Veterans	18	Improvement in depression No reduction of PTSD Sx
Shay (1991)	Fluoxetine	OT	Veterans	18	Reduced explosiveness, anger; improved mood
Shestatzky et al. (1988)	Phenelzine Placebo	DB, PC, CO	Miscellaneous PTSD	13	No difference between phenelzine and placebo
van der Kolk et al. (1994)	Fluoxetine Placebo	DB, PC	Miscellaneous PTSD	34 29	Reduction in numbing, hyperarousal & Sx of depression
Anxiolytics					
Braun et al. (1990)	Alprazolam Placebo	DB, PC	Miscellaneous PTSD	10	Modest improvement in anxiety; no effect on PTSD Sx
Loewenstein et al. (1988)	Clonazepam	OT	PTSD + MPD	5	Improved sleep, nightmares, flashbacks, and panic attacks
Risse et al. (1990)	Alprazolam	OT	Veterans	8	Severe withdrawal symptoms

Antidepressants

Mood stabilizers and others

Fesler (1991)	Valproate	OT	Veterans	16	Improved hyperarousal and hyperactivity
Lipper et al. (1986)	Carbamazepine	OT	Veterans	10	Reduction in nightmares, flashbacks, intrusion Sx; no effect on avoidance

Note. DB = double-blind; PC = placebo-controlled; CO = crossover; RA = random assignment; CR = case report; OT = open trial; Sx = symptoms; PTSD = posttraumatic stress disorder.

that effective pharmacotherapy for PTSD requires prolonged treatment; the absence of long-term studies may explain the negative results of existing inquiries. Empirical evidence supporting claims that extra time results in additional benefit for the patient is unavailable, however.

Clearly, pharmacotherapy alone is rarely sufficient to provide complete remission of PTSD (Friedman 1988). Many PTSD patients, however, find their symptoms intolerable—to the point of self-medicating with psychoactive agents, engaging in life-threatening behavior, or attempting suicide (Hendin and Haas 1991). Clinicians therefore should weigh the partial promise of pharmacotherapy for PTSD against the risks of substance abuse, violence, and suicide. Furthermore, symptom relief provided by medication may facilitate patients' participation in psychotherapy (Friedman 1988; Shalev et al. 1993a).

PSYCHOLOGICAL DIMENSIONS OF PTSD

The Behavioral Model

The behavioral view of PTSD identifies classical conditioning as the mechanism that links symptoms of PTSD to the precipitating trauma. According to this model, patients who originally react to a traumatic event (unconditioned stimulus) with fear and arousal (unconditioned response) continue to show the same response to cues (conditioned stimuli) that have been paired with the stressful exposure.

In contrast to simple conditioning, however, learned responses in PTSD do not diminish with time. Keane et al. (1985) therefore advanced a *dual-conditioning model*. In this model, the initial "simple" conditioning (resulting in avoidance of cues immediately present during the trauma) is followed by operant conditioning, in which reductions in distress and tension reward the avoidance of a variety of internal and external cues that are loosely associated with the trauma. Such rewarded avoidance prevents the extinction of the conditioned response over time and expands the avoidant behavior to secondary and tertiary cues.

One shortcoming of the behavioral model is its inability to account for the spontaneous recurrence of distressful recollections of the trauma, the state of permanent alarm typical of PTSD, and exaggerated startle responses. Foa and Rothbaum (1989) offered a *cognitive-behavioral model* that entailed an integration between meaning propositions and conditioning. They suggested that a patient's perception of controllability and predictability—and subsequent attributions of threat—are central to the development of PTSD and therefore should be addressed in therapy.

Behavior therapy. Interventions based on behavior theory are designed to undo conditioned responses to conditioning stimuli that have been paired with the trauma. Behavior therapy proceeds either by gradual reexposure (desensitization) or massive reexposure (flooding) to the conditioning stimuli; such therapy may involve either in vivo (i.e., exposure to real objects or situations) or in vitro (i.e., laboratory-based) protocols.

Four controlled studies (Boudewyns and Hyer 1990; Cooper and Clum 1989; Foa et al. 1991; Keane et al. 1989) indicated that flooding may reduce PTSD symptoms. Keane et al. (1989) found that flooding had a significant effect on reexperiencing, anxiety, and depression. Boudewyns and Hyer (1990) found that flooding improved adjustment in Vietnam veterans; they also showed that, regardless of treatment modality, clinical improvement was associated with a reduction in physiological responses to traumatic imagery. Cooper and Clum (1989) described a positive interaction between flooding and interpersonal treatment, and Foa et al. (1991) found that prolonged exposure effectively reduced PTSD symptoms in rape victims. In contrast, however, Pitman et al. (1991) reported exacerbation of depression and panic anxiety, increased alcohol consumption, and mobilization of negative appraisal during flooding therapy (Table 12–2).

Desensitization in vitro has been the object of two controlled studies (Brom et al. 1989; Peniston 1986) and several open trials (e.g., Vaughan and Tarrier 1992). Peniston (1986) found that desensitization was associated with reductions in nightmares, flashbacks, muscle tension, and readmission rates. Brom et al. (1989) compared desensitization with brief dynamic therapy, hypnosis, and waiting-list controls; all active treatment modalities resulted in measurable improvement.

Table 12–2. Psychological treatment of PTSD

Author(s)	Design	N	Population	Method/technique	Results/conclusions
Psychodynamic therapy					
Brom et al. (1989)	CT	112	Miscellaneous trauma	Compared desensitization, hypnotherapy, psychodynamic therapy, and waiting-list control	Significant improvement of treated cases across treatment modalities
Lindy (1988)	OT	21	War veterans	Intensive psychoanalytic psychotherapy	Improvement in general psychiatric symptoms, intrusion; no effect on avoidance
Cognitive therapy					
Foa et al. (1991)	CT	45	Rape victims	Compared stress inoculation training (SIT), prolonged exposure (PE), supportive counseling (SC), and wait-list control (WL)	All treatment conditions produced improvement; immediately after treatment, SIT > SC and WL; on 3.5-month follow-up, PE > all others

Resick and Schnicke (1992)	CT	19	Sexual assault	Compared cognitive processing therapy with waiting-list control	Improvement in PTSD Sx and depression in the treatment group maintained for 6 months
Exposure in Vitro: **Flooding**					
Boudewyns and Hyer (1990)	CR	51	Vietnam veterans	Compared direct therapeutic exposure (DTE) with counseling in inpatients	More Ss treated with DTE identified as treatment successes on adjustment scale scores; decreased physiological responses correlate with improvement
Cooper and Clum (1989)	CT	14	Vietnam veterans	Compared flooding and standard treatment with standard treatment alone	Flooding increased effectiveness of usual treatment on reexperiencing and sleep disturbances but had no effect on depression, anxiety, and violence-proneness

(continued)

Table 12–2.   Psychological treatment of PTSD (*continued*)

Author(s)	Design	N	Population	Method/technique	Results/conclusions
Fairbank and Keane (1982)	CT	2	War veterans	Flooding	Generalization of extinction along thematic cues; relative independence of anxiety associated with other traumatic events
Keane et al. (1989)	CT	24	Vietnam veterans	Compared flooding with waiting list	Improvement in reexperiencing, anxiety, and depression in flooding group; no effect on numbing and social avoidance
Exposure in vitro: desensitization					
Peniston (1986)	CT	16	Vietnam veterans	Desensitization assisted by biofeedback versus no treatment control	Reduction in nightmares, flashbacks, muscle tension, and readmissions rate in active treatment group
Richards and Rose (1991)	CR	4	Miscellaneous nonmilitary trauma	In vivo exposure vs. imaginal exposure	Exposure improved phobias; imaginal flooding improved Sx of dysphoria and some phobic symptoms

Study		N	Population	Treatment	Outcome
Shalev et al. (1992b)	CR	4	Miscellaneous nonmilitary trauma	Desensitization	Reduction in physiological responses specific to recollections treated with desensitization
Vaughan and Tarrier (1992)	OT	10	Miscellaneous trauma	Image habituation training	6 Ss improved; 2 showed moderate improvements, 2 showed minimal improvement
Exposure in vivo Scurfield et al. (1992)	OT	45	Vietnam veterans	Helicopter ride therapy	Increase in intrusive and painful memories following exposure, better peer group bonding; desensitization to helicopter ride
Exposure in vitro Z. Solomon et al. (1992)	CT	80	Israeli war veterans	Military fitness and training program vs. no treatment	Worsening of PTSD, psychiatric symptomatology, and social functioning immediately after treatment and 9 months later

(continued)

Table 12–2. Psychological treatment of PTSD (*continued*)

Author(s)	Design	N	Population	Method/technique	Results/conclusions
Rehabilitation and work exposure					
Grunert et al. (1992)	OT	51	Work-related hand injury	Graded work exposure	88%–92% return to work and 80%–81% working full-time on 6-month follow-up; decrease in work-avoidance in patients with flashbacks

Note. OT = open trial; CT = controlled trial; CR = case report; Sx = symptoms; Ss = subjects.

Studies evaluating the effect of behavior therapy on physiological responses to imagery of the trauma (Fairbank and Keane 1982; Shalev et al. 1992b) showed that the positive results of such treatment may not extend to traumatic experiences other than those addressed in therapy. Desensitization of one trauma (e.g., combat action, rape) may not generalize to sequences of traumatic experiences engendered by complex events (e.g., war, repeated abuse). The usefulness of behavior therapy in patients exposed to prolonged traumatization requires further study.

The largest study of exposure in vivo (Z. Solomon et al. 1992) assessed the effects of a complex rehabilitation and training program conducted by the Israel Defense Force 4 years after the Lebanon war to change the pervasive course of PTSD in veterans of that war. The program included exposure to military cues (e.g., rifle range, artillery fire) within a military milieu, along with cognitive, behavioral, and supportive interventions. The study compared 40 program participants with 40 PTSD control subjects who did not participate using measures of PTSD, general psychiatric symptomatology, self-efficacy, and social and psychological adjustment. The study also evaluated intra-individual changes induced by the program. Program participants fared worse than control subjects and worse than their own initial scores immediately and 9 months after the program.

Scurfield et al. (1992) reported similar reactivation of traumatic memories in Vietnam veterans with PTSD during "helicopter ride therapy." Exposure was associated with intrusive painful memories and in-flight reactions, but improved group cohesion produced a degree of desensitization.

In general, studies of behavioral treatment in PTSD report significant but partial improvement. Undoing of a conditioned response clearly is insufficient; this conclusion suggests that the pathophysiology of PTSD goes beyond learned conditioning. Moreover, direct exposure and flooding may result in reactivation and worsening of symptoms and behavior.

Cognitive Formulations of PTSD

The cognitive model of PTSD (e.g., Janoff-Bulman 1985; McCann and Pearlman 1992) postulates that a traumatic experience may reveal basic assumptions that normally underlie a patient's expectations, behavior, and appraisal (e.g., identity, world view, safety, trust, esteem, intimacy, power, or independence) as inaccurate, insufficient, or inadequate. Pathogenic assumptions (e.g., vulnerability, mistrust, or disempowerment) may subsequently replace previous assumptions and generalize to many areas of life. Cognitive therapists endeavor to diagnose and redress specific dysfunctional schemata and help the patient generate more functional alternatives.

Cognitive therapy.   Two controlled studies pertaining to victims of sexual assault indicated that cognitive therapy led to significant improvement. Foa et al. (1991) compared stress inoculation therapy—a treatment combining behavioral and cognitive techniques—with prolonged exposure, counseling, and waiting-list control. Stress inoculation therapy produced a significant reduction of PTSD symptoms immediately after treatment; prolonged exposure, however, showed greater efficacy in reducing PTSD symptoms at the 3-month follow-up. Resick and Schnicke (1992) compared cognitive processing therapy with waiting-list control individuals. Subjects in the treatment group improved in measures of depression and maintained the improvement for 6 months.

Psychodynamic Formulations of PTSD

Psychodynamic formulations of PTSD and its predecessor, "traumatic neurosis," are complex and multifaceted. Researchers have advanced two generic metaphors: damage to a component of the mental apparatus and incomplete processing of traumatic experiences.

Damage to mental apparatus.   Commenting on the repetitive and distressful nightmares of patients with traumatic neurosis, Freud (1920/1957) suggested that war trauma creates a breach in a hypothetical "stimulus barrier" that normally protects the mental apparatus from excessive amounts of "excitation." As a result of this structural impairment, the mental apparatus abruptly modifies its rules of action; instead of being dominated by homeostasis-based dynamics (exemplified by the "pleasure principle"), it becomes subjugated to a hypothetical "repetition compulsion"—a "primitive" and more "biological" set of functional rules. Accordingly, individuals with traumatic neuroses are captive of an endless repetition that directly represents the dynamics of the repetition compulsion. Freud's formulation involved a powerful insight: repetitive phenomena in traumatic neuroses do not necessarily constitute progress toward self-healing; they often express traumatic surrender of the psychic apparatus to a new set of rules.

Subsequent structural models have metaphorically repeated Freud's original concept. These formulations have been based on the appraisal that mental trauma alters the rules of mental functioning, rather than injecting new content to old conflicts. Current terminology refers to this alteration as "traumatized self" (e.g., Laufer 1988; Lifton 1988) or "collapse of structures" (Benyakar et al. 1989). The practical implications of such paradigms is a recognition that PTSD impairs the patient's self-healing capacity. Consequently, therapy must include ego-supportive maneuvers, address vulnerability in character structure, and involve the therapist in a role of participant, rather than observer.

The constructivist self-development model (McCann and Pearlman 1992) offered a bridge between self and cognitive psychology. According to this model, trauma affects three aspects of the self: self-capacities, or the ability to tolerate strong affect and regulate self-esteem; cognitive schemata, or beliefs and expectations about self and others; and intrusive trauma memories and related distressing affect.

Krystal's description, in survivors of massive trauma, of loss of affective modulation (Krystal 1978) was another variation on the theme of psychic damage. Krystal argued that psychological surrender—typical in situations of prolonged exposure to extreme adversity—leads to permanent impairment of the patient's affective life (e.g., inability to use subtle affective cues, loss of affective modulation). This impairment resembles alexithymia—a mental condition in which the individual is unable to recognize and use internal states of affect. Research has confirmed the presence of alexithymic traits in war veterans with PTSD (Hyer et al. 1990).

Unresolved mental processes. This psychodynamic model stems from the paradigm of loss, mourning, and grief. Citing similarities between symptoms of intrusion and avoidance observed in posttraumatic individuals and those in the early phase of normal grief—sketched by Freud (1917/1957) and described by Lindemann (1944)—Horowitz (1974) hypothesized that stress response syndrome (an early equivalent of PTSD) results from incomplete mental processing of the traumatic event.

From a practical point of view, this concept suggests that PTSD might resolve if patients were allowed to work through their experiences. Yet, the amount of arousal and panic associated with the reactivation of traumatic memories, the advent of dissociative reactions during exploration of the trauma, and the extent of psychic avoidance in some PTSD patients may make the explorative approach impractical in many cases.

Psychodynamic psychotherapy. Psychodynamic psychotherapy specifically addresses the meaning of trauma-related symptoms and behavior and the meaning of the traumatic event. The analytic therapist hopes that insights regarding the meaning of symptoms— conscious and unconscious—can help the patient master inner experiences and make the fabric of life whole again (Lindy 1993). Marmar et al. (1993) emphasized the importance of establishing a therapeutic alliance and noted the difficulties of that task, echoing the suggestion that the therapeutic alliance *is* the treatment for these patients, not just the facilitator of treatment (Haley 1974).

Most of the literature on psychodynamic therapy in PTSD consists of case reports; many of these studies emphasize theoretical and technical aspects of treatment. The aforementioned controlled study (Brom et al. 1989) compared brief dynamic psychotherapy with hypnotherapy, desensitization, and waiting-list control subjects; all active treatment groups improved significantly. In a well-documented treatment project (Lindy 1988), 21 Vietnam veterans with PTSD participated in individual psychoanalytic psychotherapy for a year. A decrease in intrusive phenomena and depression was recorded in patients who completed their treatment.

INSIGHTS FROM PSYCHOPHYSIOLOGICAL STUDIES

Medical literature has long recognized the link between posttraumatic morbidity and physiological disturbances. More than 300 years ago, Hoffer described physiological disturbances leading to marasma and death in Swiss soldiers experiencing nostalgia (see Rosen 1975). Meakins and Wilson (1918) recorded exaggerated heart rate responses in World War I veterans with "soldier's heart" exposed to gunfire and sudden sulfuric flames, and Drury (1918) described hypersensitivity to CO_2 inhalation in combat veterans with the "irritable heart of soldiers." During World War II, Kardiner (1941) ascribed the name "physioneurosis" to the condition currently known as PTSD; the cardinal features of the Kardiner's description were persistence of startle responses and irritability, proclivity to explosive reactions, fixation on the trauma, constriction of personality functioning, and atypical dream life.

Psychophysiological studies of PTSD (see Shalev and Rogel-Fuchs 1993) have evaluated responses to three types of stimuli: external cues reminiscent of the trauma, mental imagery of the trauma, and loud noises capable of generating auditory startle. These studies have assessed physiological responses through measurements of changes in heart rate (HR), blood pressure (BP), skin conductance (SC), and electromyograph (EMG) results.

Physiological Response to External Cues

The learned-conditioning paradigm underlies the use of external stimuli to elicit physiological responses in PTSD. Accordingly, physiological responses recorded during exposure to cues that remind the patient of the trauma are equivalent to conditioned responses.

Blanchard et al. (1982) compared the physiological responses to combat sounds of 11 Vietnam veterans with PTSD with those of nonveteran control subjects. The HR responses to combat sounds correctly classified 91% of the subjects with PTSD and 100% of the control subjects into their respective groups. Malloy et al. (1983) exposed combat veterans with PTSD, combat veterans without PTSD, and non-PTSD psychiatric inpatients to audiovisual presentation of combat scenes; the PTSD group showed significantly greater HR response. Blanchard et al. (1991) assessed the reliability of psychophysiological measures by comparing two large samples of Vietnam veterans and combat control subjects; a discriminant function equation derived from the first sample ($N = 104$) correctly identified 83% of the subjects in the second sample ($N = 96$).

Physiological Responses to Mental Imagery

Studies of responses to mental imagery differ from those of external cues in their use of the subjects' own recollections of the trauma as eliciting stimuli. These experiments, therefore, measure physiological responses to reminiscences.

Pitman et al. (1987) performed a series of studies of PTSD patients' responses to traumatic and nontraumatic mental images. The investigators asked subjects to listen to recorded scripts describing traumatic events—some standardized and others based on the subjects' individual experiences. Imagery of the subjects' personal incidents provoked extreme HR, EMG, and SC responses in PTSD subjects but not in combat control subjects. A discriminant function analysis based on the magnitude of these responses distinguished war veterans with PTSD from those without PTSD with a specificity of 100% and a sensitivity of 61%. Shalev et al. (1993b) replicated this method with a group of male and female survivors of nonmilitary events, with similar results.

Physiological Responses to Auditory Startle

The acoustic startle response (ASR) consists of a sequence of muscular and autonomic responses elicited by sudden, intense stimuli. Typical autonomic nervous system (ANS) responses (e.g., HR acceleration and deceleration, SC elevation) follow the muscular component of the ASR. The neuronal pathways of the ASR typically involve a small number of mediating synapses between receptor and effector and large interconnections between this primary neuronal circuit and brain areas responsible for central nervous system (CNS) activation and stimulus evaluation. The ASR is subject to habituation (a decrease in response amplitude on repeated presentation of the eliciting stimulus), sensitization, prepulse modification, and sensitivity to prior associative learning.

Increased startle response is a central feature of PTSD, and researchers have published several studies of ASR in PTSD. Butler et al. (1990), for example, found increased EMG responses to startling noise in PTSD patients, and Paige et al. (1990) found elevated HR responses in Vietnam veterans with PTSD. Ross et al. (1989) failed to find abnormal habituation of the eye-blink response to a series of loud tones in subjects with PTSD.

Shalev et al. (1992a) evaluated CNS and ANS responses to 15 consecutive 95-decibel, 1,000-Hz, pure tone stimuli. The study compared 14 patients with PTSD with 14 patients with other anxiety disorders, 19 subjects with past traumatic experiences but no current PTSD, and 15 mentally healthy subjects with no major traumatic events in their past. The SC reaction failed to habituate to consecutive presentations of auditory stimuli only in the PTSD group (Figure 12–1); 13 of 14 PTSD subjects (93%)—but only 11 of 48 control subjects (22%)—failed to reach a SC nonresponse criterion during the tone presentations ($\chi^2 = 25.6$, $P < .0001$). Subjects with PTSD also showed greater HR response.

Pitman et al. (1993) replicated these findings with 69 Vietnam veterans (37 with current PTSD, 13 with past but no current PTSD, and 19 with no past or current PTSD). Interestingly, the ASR of the 13 subjects with past history of PTSD resembled that of subjects with current PTSD, suggesting that abnormal ASR might be a trait marker rather than a state marker of the disorder.

Integration: Levels of Physiological Responses in PTSD

The coexistence of increased physiological responsiveness to external and internal cues in patients with PTSD and findings of abnormal startle response in PTSD exemplify the complexity of the disorder. Studies of physiological responses to external stimuli led Kolb and Multalipassi (1982) to hypothesize that PTSD involves a "conditioned emotional response," similar to that observed in research on fear conditioning in animals. Fear conditioning may be acquired, maintained, and mediated by mesocortical structures in the brain and modulated by cortical structures. In other words, implicit memories of trauma capable of eliciting alarm and arousal may be imprinted at lower levels of the brain.

In contrast, cortical processes involving semantic recognition and verbal interpretation mediate physiological responsiveness to verbal scripts of trauma. These responses might be considered analogous to findings of conditioned responses to cues reminiscent of trauma. This analogy suggests, however, that mental representations of trauma may constitute the equivalent of a conditioning stimulus. Pavlov's concept of a secondary system of representations (Pavlov 1927/1960)—a mental network of recollections, verbal representations, and images that, in humans, plays the role of a "second reality" and

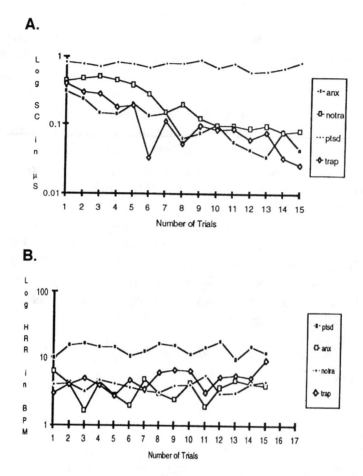

Figure 12–1.   Skin conductance (**a**) and heart rate (**b**) responses to loud tones in posttraumatic stress disorder (PTSD) and control subjects. ANX = control subjects with non-PTSD anxiety disorders; NOTRA = control subjects with no history of trauma; TRAP = control subjects with past exposure to traumatic experiences; μS = microsiemens; BPM = beats per minute. *Source.*   Shalev AY, Orr SP, Peri T, et al: "Physiologic responses to loud tones in Israeli post-traumatic stress disorder patients." Arch Gen Psychiatry 49:870–875, 1992a

is capable of reinforcing learning and conditioning in the absence of external reinforcement—exemplifies this notion.

Stimuli used to elicit startle response such as tones, white noise, or air puffs bear no associative link with traumatic events. Consequently, responses elicited by these stimuli do not reflect learned conditioning. Studies of the ASR suggest, therefore, that PTSD entails an alteration of CNS responsiveness to elementary stimuli beyond conditioned responses. The aforementioned defect in habituation also recalls the natural history of the disorder, which consists of unremitting repetition (that is, nonhabituation) of a normally self-remitting stress response (Horowitz 1974). These three modes of abnormal responses in PTSD reflect three distinct, but mutually interacting, levels of physiological activity, in which traumatic experiences affect the PTSD patient's neuronal and mental function.

LEVELS OF TRAUMA: QUESTIONS FOR THE FUTURE

Are Memories of Trauma Indelible?

Experiments on fear conditioning in animals provide a first approximation to some of the mechanisms underlying PTSD. LeDoux (1990) showed that the acquisition of the conditioned fear response in rodents is mediated by a subcortical circuit involving the sensory thalamus, as well as the lateral and subsequently the central nuclei of the amygdala. LeDoux and his colleagues further showed that although lesions of the sensory cortex do not interfere with the acquisition of emotional conditioning, such lesions prevent the extinction of fear-conditioned responses. This finding suggests that the mechanism underlying the extinction of conditioned fear responses involves cortical inhibitory control, rather than the undoing of subcortical learning. LeDoux therefore postulated that subcortical traces of fear conditioning are indelible and, by extension, that emotional memory may be forever (LeDoux 1990).

PTSD closely approximates LeDoux' proposition. Clinical features of PTSD—such as reactivation by reexposure to traumatic stressors, delayed onset, and reemergence of traumatic memories in elderly survivors faced with fatal disease or senility (Holloway and Ursano 1984; Op den Velde et al. 1993)—conform with the concept of indelible memory held under control by inhibitory cortical activity. Accordingly, clinical healing of PTSD may involve enhanced cortical control over previously acquired fear conditioning rather than elimination of traumatic memories.

The Role of the Amygdaloid Complex in PTSD

The coexistence of conditioned emotional response and abnormal startle in PTSD also conforms with the hypothesis that the mesocortical nucleus of the amygdala may play a central role in the etiology and pathophysiology of the disorder. Pitman (1989) theorized that the durability of conditioned responses in PTSD results from memory consolidation—mediated by a release of stress hormones—at the level of the amygdala. Similarly, LeDoux's (1990) model implies a role for the central and lateral nuclei of the amygdala in fear-conditioned responses.

Davis (1986, 1990) showed that lesions of the amygdala block fear-potentiated startle. Conversely, low-level electrical stimulation of the amygdala markedly increases the amplitude of the ASR, suggesting that the startle reflex is a sensitive index of amygdala stimulation. Davis subsequently suggested that the central nucleus of the amygdala plays a pivotal role in fear-potentiated startle, mediating the perceptual processes involved in the recognition of the fear signal and the startle circuit.

Finally, electrical stimulation of the amygdaloid structures during neurosurgical procedures in humans (as well as in animal experiments) produces behavioral responses that correspond with PTSD, such as apprehension, violent attack behavior, feelings of horror and fear, memory-like hallucinations, and heightened startle (Strub and Black 1988). Together, these findings assign a pivotal role to the amygdaloid structure in the pathogenesis and pathophysiology of PTSD.

TOWARD AN INTEGRATED MODEL OF PTSD

Psychiatrists should bear in mind that some of the effects of trauma might be indelible—and hence inaccessible to curative therapy. Practitioners should reconsider attempts to cure chronic cases of PTSD with heroic treatment programs (e.g., reexposure, exploratory psychotherapy) that aim to undo the etiological mechanisms of the disorder; instead, they should set more realistic goals (e.g., management of depressed mood or hyperarousal, vocational rehabilitation, family education, prevention of adverse health practices).

Grunert et al. (1992) demonstrated the promise of such an approach in a study of a graded work-exposure program. This program involved 51 patients with PTSD secondary to work-related hand injuries; 90% of these patients returned to work, including 73% of those who were experiencing flashbacks. Defining the parameters of disabilities associated with PTSD (e.g., stimulus sensitivity, reduced attention span, memory and learning impairment) is an important challenge for the future.

The evidence outlined above suggests that unidimensional formulations of PTSD offer only a partial picture of this complex condition. Freud's early homeostatic model, for example, could not account for the clinical phenomenon of distressing nightmares typical of traumatic neuroses and had to be expanded to include the new generic concepts of repetition, compulsion, and death instinct. Learning theories did not provide a satisfactory explanation for the presence of tonic arousal and the spontaneous emergence of traumatic memories in daydreams, nightmares, and flashbacks; neurobiological models fell short of providing an integrated paradigm for PTSD. Finally, no treatment modality offers adequate control of PTSD symptoms.

These shortcomings point to the need for a multidimensional approach to understanding and treating PTSD. Discontent with the therapeutic results of unidimensional treatment methods (e.g. Braun et al. 1990; Lindy 1988; Pitman et al. 1991) further attest to that need.

Shalev et al. (1993a) proposed a four-level model based on Engel's *biopsychosocial* paradigm (Engel 1980). The biological level of this model refers to neurological dysfunction; the psychological-behavioral level involves a conditioned fear response. The third level incorporates altered networks of meanings associated with the traumatic event that may be juxtaposed on earlier unconscious conflicts, and the social level includes real and symbolic interactions between the individual and society that are involved in the acquisition, maintenance, and healing of trauma. Figure 12–2 schematically presents this proposed four-level model, along with the treatment modality associated with each level (e.g., pharmacological, behavioral, psychodynamic, psychosocial). This multilevel model implies that none of these treatments should be applied in isolation.

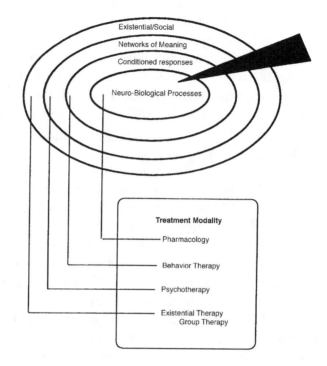

Figure 12–2. Levels of trauma: the biopsychosocial model. *Source.* Shalev AY, Galai T, Eth S: "Levels of trauma: a multidimensional approach to the treatment of PTSD." Psychiatry 6:166–177, 1993a

REFERENCES

American Psychiatric Association: Diagnostic and Statistical Manual of Mental Disorders, 3rd Edition. Washington, DC, American Psychiatric Press, 1980

American Psychiatric Association: Diagnostic and Statistical Manual of Mental Disorders, 3rd Edition, Revised. Washington, DC, American Psychiatric Press, 1987

Benyakar M, Kutz I, Dasberg H, et al: The collapse of structure: a structural approach to trauma. J Trauma Stress 2:431–450, 1989

Blanchard EB, Kolb LC, Pallmeyer TP, et al: A psychophysiological study of post traumatic stress disorder in Vietnam veterans. Psychiatr Q 54:220–229, 1982

Blanchard EB, Kolb LC, Prins A: Psychophysiological responses in the diagnosis of posttraumatic stress disorder in Vietnam veterans. J Nerv Ment Dis 179:97–101, 1991

Bleich A, Siegel B, Garb R, et al: Post-traumatic stress disorder following combat exposure: clinical features and psychopharmacological treatment. Br J Psychiatry 149:354–369, 1986

Boudewyns PA, Hyer L: Physiological response to combat memories and preliminary treatment outcome in Vietnam veterans PTSD patients treated with direct therapeutic exposure. Behavior Therapy 21:63–87, 1990

Braun P, Greenberg D, Dasberg H, et al: Core symptoms of posttraumatic stress disorder unimproved by alprazolam treatment. J Clin Psychiatry 51:236–238, 1990

Brom D, Kleber RJ, Defares PB: Brief psychotherapy for posttraumatic stress disorders. J Consult Clin Psychol 57:607–612, 1989

Butler RW, Braff DL, Rausch JL, et al: Physiological evidence of exaggerated startle response in a subgroup of Vietnam veterans with combat-related PTSD. Am J Psychiatry 147:1308–1312, 1990

Cannon WB: The Wisdom of the Body. New York, Norton, 1932

Charney DS, Dutch AY, Krystal JH, et al: Psychobiologic mechanisms of posttraumatic stress disorder. Arch Gen Psychiatry 50:294–306, 1993

Cooper NA, Clum GA: Imaginal flooding as a supplementary treatment for PTSD in combat veterans: a controlled study. Behavior Therapy 20:381–391, 1989

Davidson J: Drug therapy of post-traumatic stress disorder. Br J Psychiatry 160:309–314, 1992

Davidson J, Kudler H, Smith R, et al: Treatment of posttraumatic stress disorder with amitriptyline and placebo. Arch Gen Psychiatry 47:259–266, 1990

Davidson JR, Kudler HS, Saunders WB, et al: Predicting response to amitriptyline in posttraumatic stress disorder. Am J Psychiatry 150:1024–1029, 1993

Davis M: Pharmacological and anatomical analysis of fear conditioning using the fear potentiated startle paradigm. Behav Neurosci 100:814–824, 1986

Davis M: Neural system involved in fear-potentiated startle. Ann N Y Acad Sci 165–183, 1990

Drury AN: The percentage of carbon dioxide in the alveolar air, and the tolerance to accumulating carbon dioxide in cases so called "irritable heart of soldiers." Heart 7:165–173, 1918

Engdahl, Brian E, Speed N, et al: Comorbidity of psychiatric disorders and personality profiles of American World War II prisoners of war. J Nerv Ment Dis 179:181–187, 1991

Engel GL: The clinical application of the biopsychosocial model. Am J Psychiatry 137:535–544, 1980

Fairbank JA, Keane TM: Flooding for combat-related stress disorders: assessment of anxiety reduction across traumatic memories. Behavior Therapy 13:499–510, 1982

Fesler FA: Valproate in combat-related posttraumatic stress disorder. J Clin Psychiatry 52:361–364, 1991

Foa EB, Rothbaum BO: Behavioural psychotherapy for post-traumatic stress disorder. International Review of Psychiatry 1:219–226, 1989

Foa EB, Rothbaum BO, Riggs DS, et al: Treatment of posttraumatic stress disorder in rape victims: a comparison between cognitive-behavioral procedures and counseling. J Consult Clin Psychol 59:715–723, 1991

Freud S: Mourning and melancholia (1917), in The Standard Edition of the Complete Psychological Works of Sigmund Freud, Vol 14. Translated and edited by Strachey J. London, Hogarth Press, 1957, pp 243–258

Freud S: Beyond the pleasure principles (1920), in The Standard Edition of the Complete Psychological Works of Sigmund Freud, Vol 18. Translated and edited by Strachey J. London, Hogarth Press, 1957, p 64

Friedman MJ: Toward rational pharmacotherapy for posttraumatic stress disorder: an interim report. Am J Psychiatry 145:281–285, 1988

Grunert BK, Devine CA, Smith CJ, et al: Graded work exposure to promote work return after severe hand trauma: a replicated study. Ann Plast Surg 29:532–536, 1992

Haley S: When the patient reports atrocities. Arch Gen Psychiatry 30: 191–196, 1974

Hendin H, Haas AP: Suicide and guilt as manifestations of PTSD in Vietnam combat veterans. Am J Psychiatry 148:586–591, 1991

Holloway HC, Ursano RJ: The Vietnam veteran: memory, social context and metaphor. Psychiatry 47:103–108, 1984

Horowitz MJ: Stress response syndromes: character style and dynamic psychotherapy. Arch Gen Psychiatry 31:768–781, 1974

Hyer L, Woods M, Summers MN, et al: Alexithymia among Vietnam veterans with posttraumatic stress disorder. J Clin Psychiatry 51:243–247, 1990

Irwin M, Van-Putten T, Guze B, et al: Pharmacologic treatment of veterans with posttraumatic stress disorder and concomitant affective disorder. Ann Clin Psychiatry 1:127–130, 1989

Janoff-Bulman R: The aftermath of victimization: rebuilding shattered assumptions, in Trauma and its Wake: The Study and Treatment of Post-Traumatic Stress Disorder. Edited by Figley CR. New York, Brunner/Mazel, 1985, pp 15–36

Kardiner A: The Traumatic Neurosis of War. New York, Hoeber, 1941

Keane TM, Fairbank JA, Caddel MT, et al: A behavioral approach to assessing and treating post-traumatic stress disorders in Vietnam veterans, in Trauma and its Wake: The Study and Treatment of Post-Traumatic Stress Disorder. Edited by Figley CR. New York, Brunner/Mazel, 1985, pp 257–294

Keane TM, Fairbank JA, Caddel JM, et al: Implosive (flooding) therapy reduces symptoms of PTSD in Vietnam combat veterans. Behavior Therapy 20:245–260, 1989

Kinzie J, Leung P: Clonidine in Cambodian patients with posttraumatic stress disorder. J Nerv Ment Dis 177:546–550, 1989

Kolb LC: A neuropsychological hypothesis explaining the post-traumatic stress disorder. Am J Psychiatry 144:989–999, 1987

Kolb LC, Multalipassi LR: The conditioned emotional response: a sub-class of the chronic and delayed post-traumatic stress disorder. Psychiatric Annals 12:979–987, 1982

Kosten TR, Frank JB, Dan E, et al: Pharmacotherapy for posttraumatic stress disorder using phenelzine or imipramine. J Nerv Ment Dis 179: 366–370, 1991

Krystal H: Trauma and affect. Psychoanal Study Child 33:81–116, 1978

Krystal JH, Kosten TR, Southwick S, et al: Neurobiological aspects of PTSD: review of clinical and pre-clinical studies. Behavior Therapy 20: 177–198, 1989

Laufer RS: The serial self: war trauma, identity and adult development, in Human Adaptation to Extreme Stress from the Holocaust to Vietnam. Edited by Wilson JP, Harel Z, Kahana B. New York, Plenum, 1988, pp 33–54

LeDoux JE: Information flow from sensation to emotion: plasticity in the neural computation of stimulus value, in Learning and Computational Neuroscience: Foundation of Adaptive Networks. Edited by Gabriel M, Moore J. Cambridge, MA, Massachusetts Institute of Technology Press, 1990, pp 3–51

Lerer B, Bleich A, Kotler M, et al: Posttraumatic stress disorder in Israeli combat veterans: effect of phenelzine treatment. Arch Gen Psychiatry 44:976–981, 1987

Lifton RJ: Understanding the traumatized self: imagery symbolization and transformation, in Human Adaptation to Extreme Stress from the Holocaust to Vietnam. Edited by Wilson JP, Harel Z, Kahana B. New York, Plenum, 1988, pp 7–32

Lindemann E: Symptomatology and management of acute grief. Am J Psychiatry 101:141–148, 1944

Lindy JD: Vietnam—A Casebook. New York, Brunner/Mazel, 1988

Lindy JD: Focal psychoanalytic psychotherapy of posttraumatic stress disorder, in International Handbook of Traumatic Stress Syndromes. Edited by Wilson JP, Raphael B. New York, Plenum, 1993, pp 803–809

Lipper S, Davidson JRT, Grady TA, et al: Preliminary study of carbamazepine in posttraumatic stress disorder. Psychosomatics 72: 849–854, 1986

Loewenstein RJ, Hornstein N, Farber B: Open trial of clonazepam in the treatment of posttraumatic stress symptoms in MPD. Dissociation 1: 3–12, 1988

Malloy PE, Fairbank JA, Keane TM: Validation of a multidimensional assessment of post traumatic stress disorder in Vietnam veterans. J Consult Clin Psychol 51:488–494, 1983

Marmar CR, Foy D, Kagan B, et al: An integrated approach for treating posttraumatic stress, in American Psychiatric Press Review of Psychiatry, Vol 12. Edited by Oldham JM, Riba MB, Tasman A. Washington, DC, American Psychiatric Press, 1993, pp 239–272

Mason JW, Giller EL, Kosten TR, et al: Psychoendocrine approach to the diagnosis and pathogenesis of posttraumatic stress disorder, in Biological Assessment and Treatment of Posttraumatic Stress Disorder. Edited by Giller EL. Washington, DC, American Psychiatric Press, 1990, pp 65–87

McCann IL, Pearlman LA: Constructivist self-development theory: a theoretical framework for assessing and treating traumatized college students. J Am Coll Health 40:189–196, 1992

McFarlane AC: Multiple diagnoses in posttraumatic stress disorder in the victims of a natural disaster. J Nerv Ment Dis 180:498–504, 1992

Meakins JC, Wilson RM: The effect of certain sensory stimulations on respiratory and heart rate in cases so called "irritable heart." Heart 7: 17–22, 1918

Mellman TA, Randolph CA, Brawman-Mintzer O, et al: Phenomenology and course of psychiatric disorders associated with combat-related posttraumatic stress disorder. Am J Psychiatry 149:1568–1574, 1992

Morgan CA, Southwick S, Grillon C, et al: Yohimbine potentiates acoustic startle response in humans. Paper presented at the 6th annual meeting of the International Society for Traumatic Stress Studies, New Orleans, LA, October 1990

Nagy L, Southwick SM, Charney DS: Open prospective trial of fluoxetine for posttraumatic stress disorder. J Clin Psychopharmacol 13:107–113, 1993

Op den Velde W, Falger PRJ, de Groen JHM, et al: Posttraumatic stress disorder in Dutch resistance veterans from World War II, in International Handbook of Traumatic Stress Syndromes. Edited by Wilson JP, Raphael B. New York, Plenum, 1993, pp 219–230

Paige SR, Graham M, Reid MG, et al: Psychophysiological correlates of posttraumatic stress disorder in Vietnam veterans. Biol Psychiatry 27:419–430, 1990

Pavlov IP: Conditioned Reflexes: An Investigation of the Physiological Activity of the Cerebral Cortex (1927). Edited and translated by Anrep GV. New York, Dover, 1960

Peniston EG: EMG biofeedback assisted desensitization treatment for Vietnam combat veterans post traumatic stress disorder. Clinical Biofeedback Health 9:35–41, 1986

Pitman RK: Posttraumatic stress disorder, hormones and memory. Biol Psychiatry 26:221–223, 1989

Pitman RK: Posttraumatic obsessive compulsive disorder: a case study. Compr Psychiatry 34:102–107, 1993

Pitman RK, Orr S, Shalev A: Once bitten, twice shy. Beyond the conditioning model of PTSD. Biol Psychiatry 33:145–146, 1993

Pitman RK, Orr SP, Forgue DF, et al: Psychophysiologic assessment of posttraumatic stress disorder imagery in Vietnam combat veterans. Arch Gen Psychiatry 44:970–975, 1987

Pitman RK, van der Kolk BA, Orr SP, et al: Naloxone-reversible analgesic response to combat-related stimuli in posttraumatic stress disorder: a pilot study. Arch Gen Psychiatry 47:541–544, 1990

Pitman RK, Altman B, Greenwald E, et al: Psychiatric complications during flooding therapy for posttraumatic stress disorder. J Clin Psychiatry 52:17–20, 1991

Reist C, Kauffman CD, Haier RJ: A controlled trial of desipramine in 81 men with posttraumatic stress disorder. Am J Psychiatry 146:513–516, 1976

Resick PA, Schnicke MK: Cognitive processing therapy for sexual assault victims. J Consult Clin Psychol 60:748–756, 1992

Richards DA, Rose JS: Exposure therapy for post-traumatic stress disorder: four case studies. Br J Psychiatry 158:836–840, 1991

Risse SC, Whitters A, Burke J, et al: Severe withdrawal symptoms after discontinuation of alprazolam in eight patients with combat-induced posttraumatic stress disorder. J Clin Psychiatry 51:206–209, 1990

Rosen G: Nostalgia: a forgotten psychological disorder. Psychol Med 5:342–347, 1975

Ross RJ, Ball WA, Cohen ME, et al: Habituation of the startle reflex in posttraumatic stress disorder. J Neuropsychiatry 1:305–307, 1989

Roszell DK, McFall ME, Malas KL: Frequency of symptoms and concurrent psychiatric disorder in Vietnam veterans with chronic PTSD. Hosp Community Psychiatry 42:293–296, 1991

Scurfield RM, Wong LE, Zeerocah EB: An evaluation of the impact of "helicopter ride therapy" for in-patient Vietnam veterans with war-related PTSD. Mil Med 157:67–73, 1992

Selye H: The Stress of Life. New York, McGraw-Hill, 1956

Shalev AY, Rogel-Fuchs Y: Psychophysiology of the post-traumatic stress disorder: from sulfur fumes to behavioral genetics. Psychosom Med 55:413–423, 1993

Shalev AY, Orr SP, Peri T, et al: Physiologic responses to loud tones in Israeli post-traumatic stress disorder patients. Arch Gen Psychiatry 49:870–875, 1992a

Shalev A, Orr SP, Pitman RK: Psychophysiologic response during script driven imagery as an outcome measure in post-traumatic stress disorder. J Clin Psychiatry 53:324–326, 1992b

Shalev AY, Rogel-Fuchs Y, Pitman RK: Conditioned fear and psychological trauma. Biol Psychiatry 31:856–863, 1992c

Shalev AY, Galai T, Eth S: Levels of trauma: a multidimensional approach to the treatment of PTSD. Psychiatry 6:166–177, 1993a

Shalev A, Orr SP, Pitman RK: Psychophysiologic assessment of traumatic imagery in Israeli civilian patients with post-traumatic stress disorder. Am J Psychiatry 50:620–624, 1993b

Shay J: Fluoxetine reduces explosiveness and elevates mood on Vietnam combat vets with PTSD. J Trauma Stress 5:97–110, 1991

Shestatzky M, Greenberg D, Lerer B: A controlled trial of phenelzine in posttraumatic stress disorder. Psychiatry Res 24:149–155, 1988

Sierles CF, Chen J, McFarland RE, et al: Posttraumatic stress disorder and concurrent psychiatric illness: preliminary report. Am J Psychiatry 140:1177–1179, 1983

Solomon SD, Gerrity ET, Muff AM: Efficacy of treatment for posttraumatic stress disorder. JAMA 268:633–638, 1992

Solomon Z, Shalev AY, Spiro S, et al: The effectiveness of the Koach Project: negative psychometric outcome. J Trauma Stress 5:247–264, 1992

Strub RL, Black FW: Neurobehavioral disorders: a clinical approach, in Anatomy of Behavior. Edited by Strub RL, Black FW. Philadelphia, PA, F. A. Davis, 1988, pp 10–14

van der Kolk B, Greenberg M, Boyd H, et al: Inescapable shock, neurotransmitter and addiction to trauma: towards a psychobiology of posttraumatic stress disorder. Biol Psychiatry 22:314–325, 1985

van der Kolk BA, Dryfuss D, Michaels M, et al: Fluoxetine in posttraumatic stress disorder. J Clin Psychiatry 55:517–522, 1994

Vaughan K, Tarrier N: The use of image habituation training with post-traumatic stress disorders. Br J Psychiatry 161:658–664, 1992

Yehuda R, Giller EL, Southwick SM, et al: Hypothalamic pituitary adrenal dysfunction in posttraumatic stress disorder. Biol Psychiatry 30:1031–1048, 1993

Chapter 13

Neurobiological Alterations in PTSD: Review of the Clinical Literature

Steven M. Southwick, M.D., Rachel Yehuda, Ph.D., and Dennis S. Charney, M.D.

Health care professionals generally understand posttraumatic stress disorder (PTSD) as a psychological disorder: in response to extreme stress, an individual develops a host of reexperiencing, avoidance, and hyperarousal symptoms that the person experiences subjectively as psychological or emotional in origin. Therefore, most treatments—including individual psychotherapy, group therapy, pastoral counseling, behavior therapy, and psychoeducation—are nonorganic in nature.

In recent years, psychiatrists increasingly have recognized that they also could consider PTSD from a biological perspective. Since 1980—when DSM-III (American Psychiatric Association 1980) added the term *posttraumatic stress disorder* to the formal nosology—a series of psychophysiological, hormonal, neurotransmitter, receptor binding, electrophysiological, and brain imaging studies have begun to characterize the biological nature of this disorder. These studies strongly support the notion that severe psychological trauma can cause alterations in the patient's neurobiological response to stress, even years after the original insult, and that these longstanding alterations may contribute to a number of complaints and symptoms that patients with PTSD commonly express (Charney et al. 1993; Southwick et al. 1992).

In this chapter, we review clinical studies of neuroendocrine and neurotransmitter alterations in patients with PTSD. Although we

briefly describe preclinical, or animal, studies, we restrict our review primarily to investigations involving humans who have been
exposed to trauma. Because most published biological studies have
involved combat veterans, our analysis draws heavily on findings
from this patient population.

Preclinical studies of stress have repeatedly demonstrated alterations in multiple neuroendocrine systems; nevertheless, human
studies largely have been limited to two major neurobiological axes
of the stress response: the sympathetic nervous system (SNS) and
the hypothalamic-pituitary-adrenal (HPA) axis. Accordingly, we
emphasize these two systems in this chapter, although we mention
other systems briefly. Determining the specific behavioral effects of
a single neurotransmitter is difficult, if not impossible, because neurotransmitters interact with one another in a complex fashion. Thus,
our analysis regarding behavioral correlates of single neurotransmitter system alterations is, by definition, simplistic.

THE SYMPATHETIC NERVOUS SYSTEM

Scientists have long recognized that activation of the SNS plays an
important role in an organism's response to stressful or dangerous
situations (Cannon 1914). Although functional groups of sympathetic
fibers can fire independently, under conditions of extreme stress the
system tends to discharge as a unit to maximize mobilization and
utilization of energy. Coordinated sympathetic discharge accelerates
heart rate and increases blood pressure, allowing for greater perfu-
sion of muscles and vital organs; dilates pupils, so that more light
enters the eye; constricts skin vasculature, to limit blood loss should
injury occur; shunts blood from temporarily unnecessary splanch-
nic and renal regions to active muscle groups; and rapidly increases
energy supply to skeletal musculature by mobilizing blood glucose
and facilitating the oxidation of various food products (Gagnon 1977;
Mountcastle 1973). Widespread emergency-stimulated SNS discharge prepares the organism for what Cannon termed the "flight
or fight" response (Cannon 1914).

Psychophysiological Studies

Although stress-induced SNS activation serves a protective role in
the short run, it may result in long-term negative sequelae for some

individuals. In many individuals who develop PTSD, the SNS appears to become hyperresponsive to a host of trauma-related stimuli. The nature and extent of this hyperresponsiveness has been the subject of intense study.

In 1918, two studies described the first laboratory investigations of SNS activity among traumatized humans. Meakins and Wilson (1918) exposed combat veterans with "shell shock" to the sounds of gunfire and the smell of sulfuric flames; they found that, as a group, these veterans had greater increases in heart rate and respiratory rate than healthy control groups. Fraser and Wilson (1918) demonstrated exaggerated psychophysiological arousal—with marked increases in subjective anxiety, heart rate, and blood pressure—among war veterans, compared with healthy control subjects, in response to intravenous administration of epinephrine.

During World War II, Kardiner coined the term "physioneurosis" to describe a neurosis characterized by hypervigilance, agitation, insomnia, nightmares, and marked physiological arousal, which he believed had a profound underlying biological basis (Kardiner 1941). Grinker and Spiegel (1945) described combat soldiers who behaved as if they had an injection of adrenaline and who suffered from stimulation of the sympathetic nervous system that was chronic in nature. The belief that altered catecholamine function played a critical role in combat neurosis led some clinicians and researchers to advocate bilateral denervation of the adrenal glands as a form of treatment for highly symptomatic war veterans (Crille 1940). The first contemporary psychophysiological study demonstrated that combat sounds caused "decompensated" World War II soldiers to become more behaviorally agitated than World War II soldiers who were not described as decompensated (Dobbs and Wilson 1960).

Since 1980, researchers have conducted a series of psychophysiology studies measuring heart rate, blood pressure, and galvanic skin response at baseline and in response to trauma-related cues (e.g., Blanchard et al. 1982, 1991; Brende 1982; Malloy et al. 1983; Orr 1990; Orr et al. 1993; Pallmeyer et al. 1986; Pitman et al. 1987, 1990a; Shalev et al. 1993). These studies found marked elevations in psychophysiological parameters during provocation but few, if any, differences at baseline between combat veterans and healthy control subjects (for a comprehensive review, see Shalev and Rogel-Fuchs 1993). Researchers did not observe this hyperreactiveness in combat veterans without PTSD (Pitman et al. 1987) or in combat veterans with anxiety disorders other than PTSD (Pitman et al. 1990a)—suggesting that neither combat exposure alone nor the presence of anxiety disorders other than PTSD is sufficient to explain postwar physiological reactivity. Furthermore, psychophysiological responses to reminders of trauma also are present in civilians with PTSD (Shalev et al. 1993).

Another line of psychophysiological investigation has examined responses to auditory startle. These studies differed somewhat from the foregoing investigations in that they measured response to neutral stimuli (e.g., loud tones, air puffs, visual images) rather than trauma-related stimuli. Shalev and Rogel-Fuchs (1993) suggested that exploration of these responses in PTSD patients, compared with control subjects, would allow researchers to investigate processes that are not confounded by conscious or unconscious behaviors on the part of the subject. Indeed, these studies have provided information about processes such as habituation, learning, and extinction that researchers have hypothesized are relevant to the acquisition of symptoms following trauma and the failure to extinguish responses to reminders of the trauma.

Most of these studies (Butler et al. 1990; Kozak et al. 1988; Paige et al. 1990; Shalev et al. 1993)—although not all (Morgan et al. 1992; Ross et al. 1989)—found abnormalities in habituation in PTSD patients. McFarlane et al. (1993) demonstrated that patients with PTSD failed to differentiate between stimuli of differing relevance; they suggested that their observations were related to disturbed concentration and memory impairments in PTSD and hypothesized that a dysfunction in central noradrenergic systems mediated the observed effect.

Indeed, consistent alterations in psychophysiological responses to stress-related stimuli in humans have prompted researchers to investigate the biochemical underpinnings of SNS activation in traumatized populations. These studies have focused primarily on the three key SNS neurotransmitters: norepinephrine, epinephrine, and dopamine.

Baseline Catecholamine Studies

Twenty-four hour urine studies.   Researchers have reported that combat veteran inpatients' mean 24-hour urinary excretion of norepinephrine is elevated, compared with healthy control subjects (Yehuda et al. 1992) and psychiatric patients (Kosten et al. 1987). Pitman and Orr (1990) reported that the mean norepinephrine level in combat veterans without PTSD was statistically equivalent to that in combat veterans with PTSD, suggesting that alterations in norepinephrine excretion may be a function of trauma rather than PTSD per se. Indeed, the mean norepinephrine excretion in both groups was comparable with the level that Yehuda et al. (1992) observed for combat veterans with PTSD. Furthermore, L.M. Davidson and Baum (1986) reported elevations in resting heart rate, blood pressure, and urinary norepinephrine in residents living within 5 miles of the Three Mile Island nuclear power plant, regardless of PTSD status.

Studies of urinary epinephrine have produced less consistent results. Although Kosten et al. (1987) and Yehuda et al. (1992) reported increased levels of 24-hour urinary epinephrine excretion among inpatients with PTSD, outpatients with PTSD did not appear to have higher epinephrine excretion (Pitman and Orr 1990; Yehuda et al. 1992). Urinary dopamine excretion, however, was elevated in inpatients with PTSD and in outpatients with PTSD (Yehuda et al. 1992).

Baseline plasma studies.   Unlike 24-hour urine studies, baseline plasma norepinephrine studies generally have found no significant differences between PTSD patients and healthy control subjects. In separate studies measuring norepinephrine responses to war-related laboratory stimuli, McFall et al. (1990) and Blanchard et al. (1991) reported similar resting baseline norepinephrine values in PTSD patients and control subjects; McFall et al. (1990) also found no differences in baseline levels of plasma epinephrine. Hamner et al. (1994) measured noradrenergic responsiveness in combat veterans with PTSD following exercise stress; they also found no baseline differences between patients and control subjects. Finally, Southwick et al. (1993a) reported comparable baseline plasma levels of the major norepinephrine metabolite, 3-methoxy-4-hydroxy-phenylglycol (MHPG), prior to yohimbine infusion among PTSD patients and control subjects.

However, the only published study examining plasma levels of dopamine (Hamner et al. 1990) suggested that resting levels of that neurotransmitter may be higher in PTSD patients than in control subjects. This finding is compatible with observations of increased urinary dopamine excretion (Yehuda et al. 1992).

Receptor studies. α_2-Adrenergic receptors play a key role in translating the neurochemical message of norepinephrine and epinephrine. As such, the functional status of the α_2 receptor may provide information about the long-term effects of alterations in catecholamine neurotransmission. Two separate radioligand-binding studies—one involving combat veterans (Perry et al. 1987) and another involving traumatized children (Perry 1994)—found fewer total α_2-adrenergic receptor binding sites per platelet in subjects with PTSD than in control subjects. Perry et al. (1990) hypothesized that chronic elevation of circulating catecholamines likely causes a "downregulation" or reduced number of available receptor sites. This reduction in the number of available receptor sites may represent an adaptive response to overstimulation by the agonist.

Using an in vitro model, Perry et al. (1990) also found that high concentrations of epinephrine caused a rapid and extensive loss of receptor protein from the platelet membranes of two PTSD patients compared with two control subjects. This preliminary finding appears to be consistent with a receptor-effector system that has been taxed by excessive exposure to the agonist and becomes easily fatigued.

Lerer et al. (1987, 1990) examined adenylate cyclase activation in platelet membranes, as well as cyclic adenosine monophosphate (cAMP) signal transduction in platelet membranes and intact lymphocytes, of PTSD patients. In lymphocyte preparations, basal cAMP levels and responsiveness to isoproterenol and forskolin stimulation was lower in PTSD patients than in control subjects. These findings appear to reflect diminished responsiveness of the receptor adenylate-cyclase complex in patients with PTSD. The results of the studies by Lerer et al. (1987, 1990) and Perry et al. (1990) point to potential abnormalities at the adrenergic receptor level and at sites distal to the receptor; these findings require further clarification.

Provocation or Challenge Studies

Challenge studies are designed to evaluate biological systems under controlled conditions that intentionally provoke the system.

Under this approach, the researcher exposes the subject to external stimuli such as recorded trauma transcripts or exogenously administered biological substances, then records behavioral, physiological, and neuroendocrine responses to the provocation. The results allow the researcher to draw inferences about the functional status of the particular biological system under investigation.

McFall et al. (1990) found parallel increases and higher levels of subjective distress, blood pressure, heart rate, and plasma epinephrine in combat veterans with PTSD than in control subjects during and after a combat film but not in response to the film of an automobile accident. The parallel increases suggested that heightened physiological reactivity was related to circulating catecholamines—specifically, epinephrine—and that the heightened response was specific to trauma-related cues. Blanchard et al. (1991) reported similar changes in norepinephrine using auditory combat-related stimuli; their comparison group comprised combat veterans without PTSD.

Dinan et al. (1990) used a desipramine growth hormone challenge to probe postsynaptic α_2-adrenergic receptor function in 8 traumatized women; they found no difference between traumatized subjects with PTSD and control subjects in desipramine-stimulated growth hormone levels. Using an intravenous challenge paradigm in a 20-year-old car accident victim with PTSD, Hansenne et al. (1991) reported a blunted growth hormone response to intravenous clonidine. Researchers generally believe that the growth hormone response to clonidine is an index of noradrenergic function; blunting therefore suggests heightened noradrenergic sensitivity, along with possible downregulation of noradrenergic receptors. After successful treatment, Hansenne et al. (1991) reported a normal growth hormone response to clonidine, which they interpreted as evidence for a relationship between noradrenergic dysregulation and PTSD-specific symptoms.

Intravenous lactate infusion causes panic attacks in patients with panic disorder. Although the precise mechanism of lactate-induced anxiety and panic is unknown, researchers have suggested central noradrenergic stimulation. In a study of seven Vietnam veterans with PTSD, Rainey et al. (1987) reported panic attacks in six of the seven subjects and flashbacks in all seven; because the subjects who had lactate-induced panic attacks also met criteria for comorbid panic disorder, however, the investigators could not determine whether the responses were secondary to panic disorder, PTSD, or both.

Yohimbine offers a more direct probe of noradrenergic activity. Yohimbine is an α_2-adrenergic receptor antagonist that activates noradrenergic neurons by blocking the α_2-adrenergic autoreceptor, thereby increasing presynaptic noradrenergic release. Southwick et al. (1993a) compared responses to yohimbine in 20 Vietnam combat veterans with those in 18 control subjects. Although yohimbine acts on multiple neurotransmitter systems, at the dose employed by Southwick et al. (1993a) it primarily affects the noradrenergic system. Yohimbine produced panic attacks in 70% of patients with PTSD and flashbacks in 40% of PTSD patients; there were no yohimbine-induced panic attacks or flashbacks among the control group. Plasma MHPG following yohimbine administration was elevated more than twice as much in patients with PTSD compared with control subjects—suggesting abnormal presynaptic noradrenergic reactivity in PTSD patients.

Yohimbine did not produce similar effects in major depressive disorder, schizophrenia, obsessive-compulsive disorder, or even generalized anxiety disorder (Charney et al. 1990). Yet, it resulted in comparable behavioral and cardiovascular responses in panic disorder patients (Charney et al. 1987), suggesting that PTSD and panic disorder share a common neurobiological abnormality that is related to altered sensitivity of the noradrenergic system. Because 43% of the patients with PTSD in the Southwick et al. (1993a) study did not meet criteria for comorbid panic disorder, the presence of panic disorder could not by itself explain yohimbine-induced panic attacks. Yet 89% of patients meeting criteria for both PTSD and panic disorder had yohimbine-induced panic attacks. Comorbid panic disorder in patients with PTSD may simply reflect a more pronounced abnormality of the noradrenergic system.

In summary, baseline or resting studies generally have found no differences in plasma catecholamine levels between combat veterans with PTSD and healthy control subjects. However, most 24-hour urine studies have reported increased excretion of catecholamines, and most challenge studies have found evidence for hypersensitivity of the noradrenergic system. Although 24-hour urine studies do not involve direct laboratory provocation, they do incorporate hormonal responses to day-to-day stressors. That is, catecholamine levels in 24-hour urine samples reflect the summation of phasic physiological changes in response to meaningful stimuli, as well as tonic resting levels of autonomic arousal (Murburg 1994). The studies reviewed earlier point to increased responsiveness of the SNS that is detectable under conditions of stress in severely traumatized individuals with PTSD. These findings are consistent with data showing consistent elevations in psychophysiological reactivity to trauma-related cues in combat veterans with PTSD. Researchers have not found conclusive psychophysiological evidence of tonic or baseline elevations, however.

THE HYPOTHALAMIC-PITUITARY-ADRENAL AXIS

Selye (1956) proposed the general adaptation syndrome as an extension of Cannon's flight-or-fight response (Cannon 1914). Studies of the general adaptation syndrome focused on the pituitary-adrenocortical response to stress. In response to stress, neuropeptides and neuromodulators stimulate the release of corticotropin releasing factor (CRF), which in turn stimulates the adrenal gland to release cortisol. Selye hypothesized that the amount of cortisol released during stress provides an index of stressor severity; Mason (1968) and Mason et al. (1976) provided clear evidence for a linear relationship between cortisol release and stressor severity.

Studies of the HPA axis in PTSD, however, have provided data that are incompatible with Selye's notion of the stress response (Yehuda et al. 1993b). For example, rather than the increased cortisol levels that the theory of general adaptation might predict, PTSD patients show evidence of low cortisol levels and other HPA-axis abnormalities that suggest a heightened sensitivity of this axis to stress.

Baseline Studies

Several studies have replicated the finding of low urinary cortisol excretion in patients with PTSD compared with other psychiatric patients and healthy control subjects. Mason et al. (1986) observed lower mean 24-hour urinary cortisol excretion in nine PTSD patients than in patients in four other diagnostic groups. Similarly, Yehuda et al. (1993a) found low urinary cortisol in PTSD, compared with major depression, panic disorder, bipolar mania, and schizophrenia. Urinary cortisol excretion also was lower in inpatient and outpatient combat veterans with PTSD than in nonpsychiatric, healthy control subjects (Yehuda et al. 1990). Low urinary cortisol levels do not appear to be solely a function of exposure to trauma: Yehuda et al. (1993b, 1995) found low urinary cortisol levels in Holocaust survivors with PTSD, but not Holocaust survivors without PTSD, compared with demographically matched healthy subjects. The only other study examining 24-hour urinary cortisol excretion (Pitman and Orr 1990) reported increased urinary cortisol levels in PTSD patients; this study differed, however, in the method of urine collection, radioimmunoassay, and other variables (see Yehuda et al. 1991a).

A recent study examining the circadian release of cortisol over the 24-hour diurnal cycle further supports the theory that basal plasma cortisol release is significantly lower in patients with PTSD than patients with major depression and healthy control subjects. Yehuda et al. (in press) found that cortisol levels were significantly lower—primarily in the late evening and early morning hours—in patients with PTSD. Chronobiological analysis of raw cortisol levels using multioscillator cosinor modeling revealed a higher "signal-to-noise" ratio of cortisol release in subjects with PTSD. That is, relative to lower cortisol excretion, PTSD patients tended to show large cortisol fluctuations. The investigators interpreted these data as reflecting a more dynamic HPA axis in PTSD.

Lymphocyte glucocorticoid receptors.   Because hormones cannot exert their genomic effects unless they are bound to steroid receptors, researchers have suggested that steroid receptor binding parameters are important in interpreting studies examining basal hormone secretion. Furthermore, because lymphocytes and brain glucocorticoid receptors share similar regulatory and binding characteristics, researchers also have suggested that lymphocyte glucocorticoid receptor function reflects aspects of peripheral and central cortisol regulation (Lowy 1989; Lowy et al. 1985).

Yehuda et al. (1991b, 1993a, in press) found higher numbers of lymphocyte glucocorticoid receptors in combat veterans with PTSD than in nonpsychiatric and psychiatric comparison groups. These findings are consistent with observations of low cortisol in PTSD; low circulating levels of a hormone or neurotransmitter usually are associated with an upregulation or increased number of receptors.

Yehuda (in press) also reported that glucocorticoid receptor numbers appeared to be significantly higher in combat veterans without PTSD than in healthy control subjects. This finding suggests that trauma exposure per se may result in long-lasting changes in glucocorticoid receptors. Yet, the number of glucocorticoid receptors in combat veterans who do not meet DSM-IV diagnostic criteria for PTSD appears to be smaller than the number in combat veterans with PTSD. Future studies exploring associations among trauma exposure severity, PTSD symptoms, and glucocorticoid receptor numbers are necessary to address definitively the cause of glucocorticoid receptor alterations in persons exposed to trauma.

Provocation or Challenge Studies

Researchers have used two HPA-axis challenge paradigms to study PTSD: the dexamethasone suppression test (DST) and the corticotropin releasing factor (CRF) test. Both tests provide information about central nervous system mechanisms involved in the regulation of glucocorticoids.

DST studies. Dexamethasone is a synthetic glucocorticoid that mimics the effect of cortisol; it directly inhibits the release of CRF and adrenocorticotropic hormone (ACTH). The DST involves administration of 1 mg dexamethasone at 11:00 A.M., when normal cortisol secretion is at its nadir in the diurnal cycle. The inhibition of CRF and ACTH results in a decrease in the amount of cortisol released from the adrenal gland. Administration of dexamethasone substantially reduces cortisol secretion in healthy individuals within hours; a 1-mg dose normally suppresses plasma cortisol to a level below 5 µg/dl at 8:00 A.M., and cortisol usually remains at that level at 4:00 A.M.

Studies examining cortisol response to dexamethasone in psychiatric disorders, most notably major depressive disorder, have repeatedly found nonsuppression of cortisol in about 40%–60% of depressed patients (for a comprehensive review, see APA Task Force 1987; Carroll 1982; Carroll et al. 1981). This nonsuppression likely results from either a reduced ability of glucocorticoids to suppress the release of CRF and ACTH or adrenal cortisol hypersecretion.

Five studies have investigated cortisol response to 1 mg of dexamethasone in patients with PTSD; all reported that PTSD patients without major depression had a "normal" suppression response (Dinan et al. 1990; Halbreich et al. 1989; Kosten et al. 1990; Kudler et al. 1987; Olivera and Fero 1990). Closer examination, however, revealed that PTSD patients as a group showed an exaggerated response to dexamethasone. Yehuda et al. (1991a) conducted a meta-analysis of research on the DST in PTSD patients. They averaged the mean cortisol data across all published studies; this calculation revealed a cortisol value in nondepressed PTSD subjects of 1.74 μg/dl—a value well below the established normal threshold of 5.0 μg/dl.

Findings of cortisol suppression following administration of dexamethasone in PTSD patients with major depression are less clear. Kudler et al. (1987), for example, reported that PTSD patients with major depressive disorder showed a rate of nonsuppression comparable with the rate observed in patients with major depressive disorder without PTSD, whereas Halbreich et al. (1989) and Kosten et al. (1990) found normal responses to dexamethasone even in depressed combat veterans with PTSD.

Olivera and Fero (1990) reported a 32% rate of nonsuppression in 65 combat veterans with PTSD who met comorbid criteria for major depressive disorder, although these individuals showed normal suppression after their major depression had remitted. A study examining cortisol response to dexamethasone in eight civilian women with PTSD (Dinan et al. 1990) also found normal responses to dexamethasone. The mean 4:00 P.M. postdexamethasone cortisol values of the 73 PTSD patients with comorbid depression in these two studies were somewhat higher than those reported for PTSD patients without major depression, although still well below the 5.0 μg/dl threshold for major depression.

Most of the DST studies in PTSD patients were conducted before researchers appreciated that cortisol levels in these patients tended to be lower and the number of glucocorticoid receptors larger than in healthy subjects. Therefore, these studies were designed to test for nonsuppression in PTSD; they did not focus on the possibility of an exaggerated cortisol response, or hypersuppression, to dexamethasone. Failure to observe the classic nonsuppression response to cortisol, coupled with reported HPA-axis alterations that appeared distinct from those in depression, prompted investigators to conduct studies designed to detect potential enhanced suppression of the cortisol response to dexamethasone.

Two studies explored the issue of enhanced cortisol suppression to dexamethasone, using 0.50-mg (Yehuda et al. 1993c) and 0.25-mg (Yehuda et al. in press) doses of dexamethasone. These studies found hyperresponsiveness to low doses of dexamethasone—as reflected by significantly lower cortisol levels—in PTSD patients compared with healthy subjects. Downregulation of cytosolic lymphocyte glucocorticoid receptors accompanied enhanced suppression of cortisol (Yehuda et al. in press). Interestingly, investigators found hyperresponsiveness to dexamethasone in combat veterans with PTSD who met the diagnostic criteria for major depressive disorder (Yehuda et al. 1993c) but not in combat veterans without PTSD (Yehuda et al. in press).

Hypersuppression of cortisol following administration of dexamethasone suggests that patients with PTSD do not exhibit a "classic" stress response as defined by Selye (1956). Furthermore, researchers have not observed this hypersuppression in other psychiatric disorders; it may serve as a relatively specific marker for PTSD.

CRF studies.   The CRF challenge test measures the pituitary ACTH and adrenal cortisol response to exogenous infusion of the neuropeptide CRF. Investigators have demonstrated attenuation of the normal ACTH response to CRF in patients with major depressive disorder (Gold et al. 1985, 1986; Holsboer et al. 1985, 1986). This blunted ACTH response typically occurs in hypercortisolemic patients; researchers believe this response reflects a decreased number of pituitary CRF receptors, caused by hypothalamic CRF hypersecretion (Gold et al. 1986; Holsboer et al. 1986), and/or increased negative feedback inhibition of the pituitary secondary to abnormally high circulating cortisol levels (Lowy et al. 1985).

A single study of eight subjects with PTSD suggested that the ACTH response to CRF also was blunted (Smith et al. 1989). The attenuated ACTH response in PTSD patients, however, occurred in the presence of normal, not elevated, evening plasma cortisol levels. Thus, the response to CRF in patients with PTSD may reflect a decreased pituitary sensitivity to CRF or an enhanced effect of glu-cocorticoid negative feedback on the pituitary, rather than a decrease in the number of CRF receptors (which researchers believe occurs in major depression).

OTHER NEUROBIOLOGICAL SYSTEMS

Animal studies of stress support the notion that multiple neuro-chemical systems can become altered in animals that have been ex-posed to traumatic, uncontrollable stressors (Southwick et al. 1992). In human studies, researchers have reported changes in opiate, se-rotonin, γ-aminobutyric acid (GABA), dopamine, and other hormone systems, in addition to catecholamine and HPA-axis alterations.

Opiates

Uncontrollable stress causes an increase in endogenous opiate re-lease and a subsequent increase in analgesia (Amir et al. 1986; Hemingway and Reigle 1987; Pitman et al. 1990b). Particularly after injury, this increase in analgesia appears to be adaptive, allowing the organism to focus its attention on behaviors that are necessary for survival. In animal and human studies, administration of the opiate antagonist nalaxone blocked stress-induced analgesia (Jack-son et al. 1979; Maier 1986; Pitman et al. 1990b). Using combat films as stressors, Pitman et al. (1990b) found that stress-induced analge-sia appeared to be significantly greater among combat veterans with PTSD than among healthy control subjects, suggesting that the en-dogenous opiate system may be involved in the pathophysiology of PTSD.

Serotonin

Preclinical studies examining the response of serotonin systems to traumatic stress have produced mixed results (see Charney et al. 1993). In humans, however, serotonin appears to play an important role in the regulation of aggression, impulsivity, and mood (Yehuda et al. 1988). Aberrations in these affects and behaviors are common in traumatized individuals with PTSD, suggesting that alterations in serotonin regulation may play a role in PTSD symptom formation.

Arora et al. (1993) reported a significant decrease in platelet 5-HT uptake among PTSD patients compared with healthy subjects and PTSD patients meeting criteria for comorbid major depression. Furthermore, mCPP (a mixed 5-HT receptor agonist) appears capable of inducing flashbacks and panic attacks in a subgroup of combat veterans with PTSD, suggesting heightened sensitivity of serotonergic receptors in this subpopulation (Southwick et al., unpublished data). Evidence of the partial efficacy of serotonin re-uptake inhibitors in treating PTSD-specific symptoms (J.R.T. Davidson et al. 1991; McDougal et al. 1991; Nagy et al. 1993; Shay 1992) further supports serotonergic involvement.

Thyroid

Kosten et al. (1990) compared the thyroid-stimulating response (TSR) to thyroid-releasing hormone (TRH) in 11 PTSD patients with the TSR in 28 depressed patients. In contrast to the classic blunted TSR response exhibited by many depressed patients, four of the 11 PTSD patients showed an augmented response to TRH. Mason et al. (1989) reported elevated thyroid levels in patients with PTSD compared with patients in several other diagnostic groups. More recently, Mason et al. 1994 found elevations of serum total triiodothyronine (T3) in a sample of combat veterans with PTSD ($N = 96$); they also observed increased levels of free T3, total thyroxine (T4), and thyroid-binding globuine (TBG). Free T4 levels were not elevated, suggesting that PTSD may involve increased peripheral conversion of T4 to T3 and increased thyroid hormone binding. The authors hypothesized that disturbances in the noradrenergic system underlie these thyroid disturbances.

Testosterone

Mason et al. (1990) found substantially higher serum testosterone concentrations in patients with PTSD than in patients with major depressive disorder, patients with bipolar disorder, and healthy subjects; testosterone levels in PTSD patients were comparable with those in schizophrenic patients. Although the clinical characteristics of these findings must be explored, the data lend further support to the neuroendocrine distinctiveness of PTSD and major depressive disorder.

SUMMARY

The studies we have reviewed in this chapter provide evidence for at least two relatively consistent neurobiological alterations in chronic PTSD. First, findings from psychophysiological, hormonal, receptor binding, and intravenous challenge studies have demonstrated repeatedly that reminders of the original trauma provoke hyperresponsiveness of the SNS in patients with PTSD (although studies of resting or baseline SNS activity have shown no consistent differences between patients with PTSD and control subjects). Researchers have examined a variety of parameters of altered SNS hypersensitivity, including blood pressure, pulse, plasma and urine norepinephrine and epinephrine, and plasma MHPG. Second, findings of HPA-axis alterations in PTSD suggest increased responsiveness of this system as well. Low baseline cortisol, coupled with heightened response to exogenous dexamethasone, is consistent with an HPA axis that is extremely sensitive to stress hormones. A recent chronobiological analysis of diurnal cortisol metabolism supports a mathematically derived model of enhanced signal-to-noise in the HPA axis among combat veterans with PTSD; this analysis offers further evidence of increased sensitivity.

These findings are consistent with a behavioral sensitization model of PTSD. Behavioral sensitization refers to an increased magnitude of response following repeated presentations of a particular stimulus. In this paradigm, following a stressful event, physiologic, biochemical, and behavioral responses to subsequent stressors increase over time. For example, dopamine-hydroxylase activity, tyrosine hydroxylase, and synaptic levels of norepinephrine all increase in animals exposed to repeated shock (Irwin et al. 1986; Karmarcy et al. 1984; Melia et al. 1991). When these repeatedly shocked animals subsequently are exposed to a limited shock, they respond as if the shock were much greater, by releasing an amount of norepinephrine that is appropriate for a much larger stressor. Over time, therefore, repetitive stress appears to cause a compensatory increase in norepinephrine synthesis and subsequent release.

Laboratory-induced behavioral sensitization and PTSD exhibit a number of parallels. In both cases, prior exposure to stressors may increase subsequent responses to stressors depending on variables such as dose, as well as frequency and intermittency of exposure (Antelman 1988; Post 1992; Post and Contel 1983). Animals that receive a large initial dose of cocaine, for example, show greater response on reexposure than animals that receive a small initial dose (Weiss et al. 1989). Similarly, in traumatized humans, the magnitude of combat exposure is positively correlated with the development of PTSD (Kulka et al. 1990; Southwick et al. 1993b), and prior exposure to childhood trauma—particularly trauma that is repetitive in nature—may increase the likelihood of PTSD symptoms (Bremner et al. 1993; Putnam 1993). A study of Israeli combat soldiers who fought in two successive wars, for example, found that soldiers were more likely to develop symptoms during the second war if they had suffered acute combat stress during the first war (Solomon et al. 1987).

For many patients with PTSD, symptoms do not diminish over time; instead, they increase in magnitude. Archibald and Tuddenham (1965) studied World War II veterans 20 years after the war; patients with PTSD reported increases in symptoms with the passage of time. Similarly, animal studies of behavioral sensitization and "time dependent change" (Antelman and Yehuda 1994) show that stressors can cause long-lasting and gradually increasing changes in behavioral and physiological responses to subsequent stressors.

Some researchers have advanced other neurobiological models to explain certain aspects of PTSD. These alternative paradigms include fear conditioning (Davis 1986; LeDoux 1990), overconsolidation of memory (McGaugh 1990; Pitman 1989), and failure of extinction (LeDoux 1990; Shalev and Rogel-Fuchs 1993).

Fear conditioning refers to the pairing or association of a wide variety of neutral stimuli that are present at the time of a trauma with feelings of terror and extreme anxiety evoked by the trauma (Davis 1986; LeDoux 1990). Fear conditioning causes these previously neutral stimuli to evoke similar feelings of terror. For example, the smell of burning firewood—a neutral stimulus—can act as a conditioned stimulus for an individual who has lived through a life-threatening fire. After the life-threatening fire, the smell of burning wood no longer elicits feelings of comfort and peace; instead, it evokes fear and terror. Kolb and Multalipassi (1982) termed this association the "conditioned emotional response."

Overconsolidation of memory is a process that is relatively indelible in nature; it may be established via thalamo-amygdala pathways during states of high emotion, such as fear or danger. Researchers have postulated that multiple neuromodulators—including norepinephrine, epinephrine, and opioid peptides—released in high concentrations during situations of fear contribute to overconsolidation of memory, which subsequently causes patients to reexperience symptoms such as flashbacks and nightmares (Pitman 1989). Alternatively, increased neuromodulator release at the time of the trauma may be related to the subsequent distress individuals feel when they are reminded of the original trauma.

Conditioned emotional responses usually diminish in intensity following repeated presentations of fear-conditioned stimuli, in the absence of traumatic stimuli. Researchers have suggested that the intransigence of PTSD symptomatology relates to a failure to extinguish conditioned emotional responses. *Failure of extinction* refers to a potential deficit in neuromechanisms involved in response reduction following repeated presentations of a fear-conditioned stimulus in the absence of a contiguous traumatic event (Charney et al. 1993).

Researchers have not demonstrated the applicability of such animal models of stress to PTSD (Yehuda and Antelman 1993). Although empirical research with human subjects has not yet established how these paradigms relate to PTSD, such models may be useful heuristic tools for understanding discrete aspects of human responses to trauma.

CONCLUSION

The foregoing review suggests that some aspects of PTSD are neurobiologically mediated, at least in part. In this chapter, we highlight recent advances in psychophysiological, hormone, and receptor assay methodology. As methodology in areas such as brain scanning becomes increasingly refined, researchers soon may be able to delineate more accurately the acute and long-term stress-induced changes in central and peripheral nervous system functioning. Clearer understanding of biological pathophysiology should enable psychiatrists to develop more specific and effective treatments for PTSD.

REFERENCES

American Psychiatric Association: Diagnostic and Statistical Manual of Mental Disorders, 3rd Edition. Washington, DC, American Psychiatric Association, 1980

American Psychiatric Association (APA) Task Force on Laboratory Tests in Psychiatry: The dexamethasone suppression test: an overview of its current status in psychiatry. Am J Psychiatry 144:1253–1262, 1987

Amir S, Brown ZA, Arnit A: The role of endorphins in stress: evidence and speculations. Neuroscience and Biobehavioral Research 4:77–86, 1986

Antelman SM: Time-dependent sensitization as the cornerstone for a new approach to pharmacotherapy: drugs as foreign or stressful stimuli. Drug Development Research 4:1–30, 1988

Antelman SM, Yehuda R: Time-dependent change following acute stress: relevance to the chronic and delayed aspects of PTSD, in Catecholamine Function in PTSD: Emerging Concepts. Edited by Murburg MM. Washington, DC, American Psychiatric Press, 1994, pp 87–98

Archibald HC, Tuddenham RO: Persistent stress reaction after combat: a twenty-year follow-up. Arch Gen Psychiatry 12:475–481, 1965

Arora RC, Fitchner CG, O'Connor F: Paroxetine binding in the blood platelets of posttraumatic stress disordered patients. Life Sci 53:919–928, 1993

Blanchard EB, Kolb LC, Pallmeyer TP, et al: A psychophysiological study of posttraumatic stress disorder in Vietnam veterans. Psychiatr Q 54:220–229, 1982

Blanchard EB, Kolb LC, Prins A, et al: Changes in plasma norepinephrine to combat-related stimuli among Vietnam veterans with posttraumatic stress disorder. J Nerv Ment Dis 179:371–373, 1991

Bremner JD, Southwick SM, Johnson DR, et al: Childhood abuse in combat-related posttraumatic stress disorder. Am J Psychiatry 150: 235–239, 1993

Brende JO: Electrodermal responses in post-traumatic syndromes. J Nerv Ment Dis 170:352–361, 1982

Butler RW, Braff DL, Raush JL, et al: Physiological evidence of exaggerated startle response in a subgroup of Vietnam veterans with combat-related PTSD. Am J Psychiatry 147:1308–1312, 1990

Cannon WB: Emergency function of adrenal medulla in pain and the major emotions. Am J Physiol 3:356–372, 1914

Carroll BJ: The dexamethasone suppression test for melancholia. Br J Psychiatry 140:292–304, 1982

Carroll BJ, Feinberg M, Gredan JF, et al: A specific laboratory test for the diagnosis of melancholia. Arch Gen Psychiatry 38:15–22, 1981

Charney DS, Woods SW, Goodman WK, et al: Neurobiological mechanisms of panic anxiety: biochemical and behavioral correlates of yohimbine-induced panic attacks. Am J Psychiatry 144:1030–1036, 1987

Charney DS, Woods SW, Price LH, et al: Noradrenergic dysregulation in panic disorder, in Neurobiology of Panic Disorder. Edited by Ballenger JC. New York, Wiley, 1990, pp 91–105

Charney DS, Deutch A, Krystal J, et al: Psychobiology mechanisms of posttraumatic stress disorder. Arch Gen Psychiatry 50:294–305, 1993

Crille G: Results of 152 denervations of the adrenal glands in the treatment of neurocirculatory asthenia. Military Surgeon 87:509–513, 1940

Davidson JRT, Ross S, Newman E: Fluoxetine in posttraumatic stress disorder. J Trauma Stress 4:419–423, 1991

Davidson LM, Baum A: Chronic stress and posttraumatic stress disorder. J Consult Clin Psychol 54:303–308, 1986

Davis M: Pharmacological and anatomical analysis of fear conditioning using the fear-potentiated startle paradigm. Behav Neurosci 100: 814–824, 1986

Dinan TG, Barry S, Yatham LN, et al: A pilot study of neuroendocrine test battery in posttraumatic stress. Biol Psychiatry 28:665–672, 1990

Dobbs D, Wilson WP: Observations on the persistence of neurosis. Dis Nerv Syst 21:40–46, 1960

Fraser F, Wilson EM: The sympathetic nervous system and the "irritable heart of soldiers." BMJ 2:27–29, 1918

Gagnon WF: The Nervous System. Los Altos, CA, Lange Publishing, 1977

Gold PW, Chrousos GP: Clinical studies with corticotropin releasing factor: implications for the diagnosis and pathophysiology of depression, Cushing's disease and adrenal insufficiency. Psychoneuroendocrinology 10:401–420, 1985

Gold PW, Loriaux DL, Roy A: Responses to corticotropin-releasing hormone in the hypercortisolism of depression and Cushing's disease. N Engl J Med 314:1329–1335, 1986

Grinker RR, Spiegel JP: Men Under Stress. Philadelphia, PA, Blakiston, 1945

Halbreich U, Olympia J, Carson S, et al: Hypothalamo-pituitary-adrenal activity in endogenously depressed post-traumatic disorder patients. Psychoneuroendocrinology 14:365–370, 1989

Hamner MB, Diamond BI, Hitri A: Plasma dopamine and prolactin levels in PTSD (abstract). Biol Psychiatry 27:72A, 1990

Hamner MB, Diamond BI, Hitri A: Plasma norepinephrine and MHPG responses to exercise stress in PTSD, in Catecholamine Function in Posttraumatic Stress Disorder: Emerging Concepts. Edited by Murburg MM. Washington, DC, American Psychiatric Press, 1994, pp 221–232

Hansenne M, Pitchot W, Anseau M: The clonidine test in posttraumatic stress disorder. Am J Psychiatry 148:810–811, 1991

Hemingway RB, Reigle TG: The involvement of endogenous opiate systems in learned helplessness and stress-induced analgesia. Psychopharmacology 3:353–357, 1987

Holsboer F, Gerken A, Stalla GK, et al: ACTH, cortisol and corticosterone output after ovine corticotropin-releasing factor challenge during depression and after recovery. Biol Psychiatry 20:276–286, 1985

Holsboer F, Gerken A, von Bardelenben U: Human corticotropin-releasing hormone in depression: correlation with thyrotropin secretion following thyrotropin releasing hormone. Biol Psychiatry 21:601–611, 1986

Irwin J, Ahluwalia P, Anismar H: Sensitization of norepinephrine activity following acute and chronic footshock. Brain Res 379:98–103, 1986

Jackson RL, Maier SF, Coon DI: Long-term analgesic effects of inescapable shock and learned helplessness. Science 206:91–93, 1979

Kardiner A: The traumatic neuroses of war, in Psychosomatic Medicine Monograph I-II. Washington, DC, National Research Council, 1941

Karmarcy NR, Delaney RL, Dunn AL: Footshock treatment activates catecholamine synthesis in slices of mouse brain regions. Brain Res 290:311–319, 1984

Kolb LC, Multalipassi LR: The conditioned emotional response: a sub-class of the chronic and delayed posttraumatic stress disorder. Psychiatric Annals 12:979–987, 1982

Kosten TR, Mason JW, Giller EL, et al: Sustained urinary norepinephrine and epinephrine elevation in post-traumatic stress disorder. Psychoneuroendocrinology 12:13–20, 1987

Kosten TR, Wahby V, Giller E, et al: The dexamethasone test and TRH stimulation test in post-traumatic stress disorder. Biol Psychiatry 28:657–664, 1990

Kozak MJ, Foa EB, Olasov B, et al: Psychophysiological responses of rape victims during imagery of rape and neutral scenes. Paper presented at the World Congress on Behavior Therapy. Edinburgh, Scotland, October 1988. Cited in Shalev and Rogel-Fuchs (1994)

Kudler H, Davidson J, Meador K, et al: The DST and post-traumatic stress disorder. Am J Psychiatry 144:1068–1071, 1987

Kulka RA, Schlenger WE, Fairbank JA, et al: Report of Findings from the National Vietnam Veterans Readjustment Study. New York, Brunner / Mazel, 1990

LeDoux JE: Information flow from sensation to emotion: plasticity of the neural computation of stimulus value, in Learning Computational Neuroscience: Foundations of Adaptive Networks. Edited by Gabriel M, Moore J. Cambridge, MA, MIT Press, 1990

Lerer B, Ebstein RP, Shestatsky M, et al: Cyclic AMP signal transduction in post-traumatic stress disorder. Am J Psychiatry 144:1324–1327, 1987

Lerer B, Bleich A, Bennett ER, et al: Platelet adenylate cyclase and phospholipase C activity in posttraumatic stress disorder. Biol Psychiatry 27:735–740, 1990

Lowy MT: Quantification of Type I and II adrenal steroid receptors in neuronal, lymphoid, and pituitary tissues. Brain Res 503:191–197, 1989

Lowy MT, Reder AT, Antel J, et al: Glucocorticoid resistance in depression: the dexamethasone suppression test and lymphocyte sensitivity to dexamethasone. Am J Psychiatry 141:1365–1370, 1985

Maier SF: Stressor controllability and stress-induced analgesia. Ann NY Acad Sci 467:55–72, 1986

Malloy PF, Fairbank JA, Keane TM: Validation of a multimethod assessment of posttraumatic stress disorders in Vietnam veterans. J Consult Clin Psychol 51:488–494, 1983

Mason JW: A review of psychoendocrine research on the sympathetic-adrenal medullary system. Psychosom Med 30:631–653, 1968

Mason JW, Maher JT, Hartley LH, et al: Selectivity of corticosteroid and catecholamine responses to various natural stimuli, in Psychopathology of Human Adaptation. Edited by Serban G. New York, Plenum, 1976, pp 147–171

Mason JW, Giller EL, Kosten TR, et al: Urinary free-cortisol levels in posttraumatic stress disorder patients. J Nerv Ment Dis 174:145–159, 1986

Mason JW, Kennedy JL, Kosten TR, et al: Serum thyroxine levels in schizophrenic and affective disorder diagnostic subgroups. J Nerv Ment Dis 177:351–358, 1989

Mason JW, Giller EL, Kosten TR, et al: Serum testosterone levels in posttraumatic stress disorder inpatients. J Trauma Stress 3:449–457, 1990

Mason JW, Southwick SM, Yehuda R, et al: Elevation of serum free triiodothyronine, thyroxin binding globulin and total thyroxin levels in combat related posttraumatic stress disorder. Arch Gen Psychiatry 57:629–642, 1994

McDougal C, Southwick SM, Charney DS, et al: An open trial of fluoxetine in the treatment of posttraumatic stress disorder. J Clin Psychopharmacol 1:325–327, 1991

McFall M, Murburg M, Ko G, et al: Autonomic response to stress in Vietnam combat veterans with post-traumatic stress disorder. Biol Psychiatry 27:1165–1175, 1990

McFarlane AC, Weber DL, Clark R: Abnormal stimulus processing in post-traumatic stress disorder. Biol Psychiatry 34:311–320, 1993

McGaugh JL: Significance and remembrance: the role of neuromodulatory systems. Psychological Science 1:15–25, 1990

Meakins JC, Wilson RM: The effect of certain sensory stimulation on the respiratory rate in cases of so-called "irritable heart." Heart 7:17–22, 1918

Melia KR, Nestler EJ, Haycock J, et al: Regulation of tyrosine hydroxylase (TH) in the locus coeruleus (LC) by corticotropin-releasing factor (CRF): relation to stress and depression (abstract). Neuroscience Abstracts 16:444, 1991

Morgan A, Southwick S, Grillon C, et al: Yohimbine potentiates startle reflex in humans. American Psychiatric Association 144th Annual Meeting, New Research Abstracts, Washington, DC: American Psychiatric Association, 127, 1991

Mountcastle ZB: Medical Physiology, 13th Edition. New York, CV Mosby, 1973

Murburg MM (ed): Catecholamine Function in Posttraumatic Stress Disorder: Emerging Concepts. Washington, DC, American Psychiatric Press, 1994

Nagy LM, Morgan CA, Southwick SM, et al: Open prospective trial of fluoxetine for posttraumatic stress disorder. J Clin Psychopharmacol 13:107–113, 1993

Olivera AA, Fero D: Affective disorders, DST, and treatment in PTSD patients: clinical observations. J Trauma Stress 3:407–414, 1990

Orr SP: Psychophysiologic studies of posttraumatic stress disorder, in Biological Assessment and Treatment of Post-Traumatic Stress Disorder. Edited by Giller EL. Washington, DC, American Psychiatric Press, 1990, pp 135–157

Orr SP, Pitman RK, Lasko NB, et al: Psychophysiological assessment of posttraumatic stress disorder imagery in World War II and Korean combat veterans. J Abnorm Psychol 102:152–159, 1993

Paige S, Reid G, Allen M: Psychophysiological correlates of posttraumatic stress disorders. Biol Psychiatry 27:419–430, 1990

Pallmeyer TP, Blanchard EB, Kolb LC: The psychophysiology of combat-induced posttraumatic stress disorder in Vietnam veterans. Behav Res Ther 24:645–652, 1986

Perry BD: Neurobiological sequelae of childhood trauma: PTSD in children, in Catecholamine Function in Posttraumatic Stress Disorder: Emerging Concepts. Edited by Murburg MM. Washington, DC, American Psychiatric Press, 1994, pp 131–158

Perry BD, Giller EL, Southwick SM: Altered platelet α_2 adrenergic binding sites in post-traumatic stress disorder. Am J Psychiatry 144:1511–1512, 1987

Perry BD, Southwick SM, Yehuda R, et al: Adrenergic receptor regulation in post-traumatic stress disorder, in Biological Assessment and Treatment of Post-traumatic Stress Disorder. Edited by Giller EL. Washington, DC, American Psychiatric Press, 1990, pp 87–114

Pitman RK: Posttraumatic stress disorder, hormone, and memory (editorial). Biol Psychiatry 26:221–223, 1989

Pitman R, Orr S: Twenty-four hour urinary cortisol and catecholamine excretion in combat-related posttraumatic stress disorder. Biol Psychiatry 27:245–247, 1990

Pitman RK, Orr SP, Forgue DF, et al: Psychophysiologic assessment of posttraumatic stress disorder imagery in Vietnam combat veterans. Arch Gen Psychiatry 44:970–975, 1987

Pitman RK, Orr SP, Forgue DF, et al: Psychophysiologic responses to combat imagery of Vietnam veterans with posttraumatic stress disorder versus other anxiety disorders. J Abnorm Psychol 99:49–54, 1990a

Pitman RK, van der Kolk BA, Orr SP, et al: Naloxone-reversible analgesic response to combat-related stimuli in posttraumatic stress disorder. Arch Gen Psychiatry 47:541–544, 1990b

Post RM: Transduction of psychosocial stress into the neurobiology of recurrent affect disorder. Am J Psychiatry 149:999–1010, 1992

Post RM, Contel NR: Human and animal studies of cocaine: implications for development of behavioral pathology, in Stimulants: Neurochemical, Behavioral, and Clinical Perspectives. Edited by Creese I. New York, Raven, 1983, pp 169–203

Putnam FW: Dissociative disorders in children: behavioral profiles and problems. Child Abuse Neglect 17:39–45, 1993

Rainey JM, Aleem A, Ortiz A, et al: A laboratory procedure for the induction of flashbacks. Am J Psychiatry 144:1317–1319, 1987

Ross RJ, Bell WA, Cohen ME, et al: Habituation of the startle reflex in posttraumatic stress disorder. J Neuropsychiatry 1:305–307, 1989

Selye H. The Stress of Life. New York, McGraw-Hill, 1956

Shalev AY, Rogel-Fuchs Y: Psychophysiology of the posttraumatic stress disorder: from sulfur fumes to behavioral genetics. Psychosom Med 55:413–423, 1993

Shalev AY, Orr FP, Pitman RK: Psychophysiologic assessment of traumatic imagery in Israeli civilian patients with posttraumatic stress disorders. Am J Psychiatry 150:620–624, 1993

Shay J: Fluoxetine reduces explosiveness and elevates moods in Vietnam combat vets with PTSD. J Trauma Stress 5:97–102, 1992

Smith MA, Davidson J, Ritchie JC, et al: The corticotropin releasing hormone test in patients with posttraumatic stress disorder. Biol Psychiatry 26:349–355, 1989

Solomon Z, Mikulincer M, Jakob BR: Exposure to recurrent combat stress: combat stress reactions among Israeli soldiers in the Lebanon war. Psychol Med 17:433–440, 1987

Southwick SM, Krystal JH, Johnson DR, et al: Neurobiology of posttraumatic stress disorder, in Annual Review of Psychiatry, Vol 11. Edited by Tasman A. Washington, DC, American Psychiatric Press, 1992, pp 347–367

Southwick SM, Krystal JH, Morgan AC, et al: Abnormal noradrenergic function in posttraumatic stress disorder. Arch Gen Psychiatry 50:266–274, 1993a

Southwick SM, Morgan CA, Nagy LM, et al: Trauma-related symptomatology in Desert Storm veterans: a preliminary report. Am J Psychiatry 150:1524–1528, 1993b

Weiss SRB, Post RM, Pert A, et al: Context-dependent cocaine sensitization: differential effect of haloperidol on development versus expression. Pharmacol Biochem Behav 34:655–661, 1989

Yehuda R, Antelman S: Criteria for rationally evaluating animal models of posttraumatic stress disorder. Biol Psychiatry 33:479–486, 1993

Yehuda R, Southwick SM, Mason JW, et al: Neuroendocrine aspects of suicidality. Endocrinol Metab Clin North Am 17:83–102, 1988

Yehuda R, Southwick SM, Nussbaum G, et al: Low urinary cortisol excretion in patients with PTSD. J Nerv Ment Dis 178:366–369, 1990

Yehuda R, Giller EL, Southwick SM, et al: Hypothalamic-pituitary-adrenal dysfunction in post-traumatic stress disorder. Biol Psychiatry 30: 1031–1048, 1991a

Yehuda R, Lowy MT, Southwick SM, et al: Increased number of glucocorticoid receptors in posttraumatic stress disorder. Am J Psychiatry 144: 499–504, 1991b

Yehuda R, Southwick SM, Giller EL, et al: Urinary catecholamine excretion and severity of PTSD symptoms in Vietnam combat veterans. J Nerv Ment Dis 180:321–325, 1992

Yehuda R, Boisoneau D, Mason JW, et al: Relationship between lymphocyte glucocorticoid receptor number and urinary-free cortisol excretion in mood, anxiety, and psychotic disorder. Biol Psychiatry 34: 18–25, 1993a

Yehuda R, Resnick H, Kahana B, et al: Persistent hormonal alterations following extreme stress in humans: adaptive or maladaptive? Psychosom Med 55:287–297, 1993b

Yehuda R, Southwick SM, Krystal JH: Enhanced suppression of cortisol following dexamethasone administration in posttraumatic stress disorder. Am J Psychiatry 150:83–86, 1993c

Yehuda R, Kahana B, Binder-Byrnes K, et al: Low urinary cortisol excretion in Holocaust survivors with posttraumatic stress disorder. Am J Psychiatry 152:982–986, 1995

Yehuda R, Boisoneau D, Lowy MT, et al: Dose-response changes in plasma cortisol and lymphocyte glucocorticoid receptors following dexamethasone administration in combat veterans with and without posttraumatic stress disorder. Arch Gen Psychiatry 52:583–593, 1995

Yehuda R, Teicher MH, Levengood RA, et al: Circadian regulation of basal cortisol levels in posttraumatic stress disorder, in Corticosteroid Receptors Mechanisms. Edited by deKloet C. New York, New York Academy of Sciences (in press)

Part IV

Conclusions

Chapter 14

Trauma, Time, and Recovery

Robert J. Ursano, M.D., and Carol S. Fullerton, Ph.D.

The study of psychiatric responses to trauma requires the wide-angle and the oil-immersion lenses of the profession's scientific and clinical skills. Psychiatric responses to traumatic events often exhibit more variety than practitioners may appreciate (see Table 14–1).

Psychiatric responses to trauma may comprise short-term effects, or they may extend for decades (see Chapter 8) and include increased long-term morbidity (see Chapter 10). Acute and chronic depression clearly are major concerns in the traumatic stress of civilian populations (see Chapter 5). Moreover, these effects extend beyond primary victims to disaster workers (see Chapter 3) and their families (see Chapter 4).

Comprehensive assessment of trauma and disaster victims must include identification of biological, psychological, and social impairments. Psychiatrists must assess posttraumatic stress disorder (PTSD), acute stress disorder, depression, and substance abuse, as well as psychological responses to injury (including organic brain syndromes) and social impairments that can accompany traumatic events (e.g., loss of home, school, family violence), to develop effective intervention and treatment plans. Practitioners must direct particular attention to patients who are injured in a disaster or traumatic event; almost all studies indicate that these individuals are at high risk for psychiatric illness.

The chronic stress of a disaster also may present as somatization, demoralization, or family violence. Primary care providers must be alert to these presentations and assess patients for requisite psychiatric treatment; they should avoid instituting inappropriate physical treatments when the underlying problem is anxiety, depression, or family distress.

269

Table 14–1. Psychiatric responses to trauma and disaster

Psychiatric disorders
Acute stress disorder
Posttraumatic stress disorder
Major depression
Generalized anxiety disorder
Substance abuse
Adjustment disorder
Psychological factors affecting medical condition
Hypochondrias
Organic brain syndromes
Factors affecting disease onset and recovery
Injury
Loss of property/home
Loss of job
Family stress/violence
Loss of community: school system, medical care system, police

Preventive medicine offers the best paradigm for psychiatric intervention after traumatic events and disasters. This perspective includes primary prevention (prevention of disease onset), secondary prevention (early treatment), and tertiary prevention (rehabilitation) (see Table 14–2).

Identification of high-risk groups, initial intervention to limit secondary exposure, and enhancement of the safety, predictability, and physical resources of the recovery environment are critical. Provision of rest, respite, sleep, physiological refueling (food, water), and safety are the first psychiatric interventions after most traumatic events.

Disaster workers can implement primary prevention. Informing trauma survivors about expected stressors, providing them with skills that help them develop a sense of control and mastery, and educating them about the importance of maintaining sleep/rest cycles and limiting exposure may decrease psychiatric distress. Empirical study of such preventive techniques is essential.

Table 14–2. Psychiatric intervention after trauma: preventive medicine

Primary prevention

Education about the expected

Training to develop mastery and control

Limit exposure

Sleep hygiene

Rest and maintains physiologic needs

Education of spouse/significant others to encourage "natural debriefing"

Secondary prevention

Restore safety and community services

Educate primary care providers

Triage

Outreach to injured for early diagnosis

Recognition of somatization as possible psychiatric distress

Educate teachers in early detection of distress

Debriefing

Psychotherapy and appropriate medication

Tertiary prevention

Treatment of comorbid disorders

Alertness to family distress of chronic loss and demoralization, spouse and child abuse

Compensation

Counteracting withdrawal and social detachment

Psychotherapy and appropriate medication

Debriefing is an aspect of secondary prevention (early treatment). Although debriefing is common, it is neither well defined nor well studied. Its use prior to reestablishment of a safe environment and a return to physiological balance (sleep, food, water) may be useless at best; at worst, it may further impair the patient's cognitive integration of the traumatic event.

Traumatic events may include a variety of stressors: life threat, traumatic bereavement, exposure to the grotesque, traumatic loss of property, and threat to loved ones. The California firestorms, Hurricane Andrew, and the Vietnam War and Persian Gulf War—all highlighted in this volume—are examples of multiple-stressor traumatic events. Such events involve several traumatic stressors; they extend for weeks and months, not moments. This pattern characterizes most disaster events, including many traumatic events that appear initially to involve single stressors.

To discern the effects of trauma, psychiatrists must understand these multievent traumas; also, researchers must seek opportunities to examine single-trauma exposures that are not confounded by the multiple stressors of disaster events (e.g., exposure to the grotesque in body handlers, the effects of indirect exposure in spouses and significant others of disaster workers). Studies of multievent and single-exposure traumas can complement each other and greatly aid psychiatry's understanding of the complexity of traumatic stress.

Researchers have only recently begun to examine trauma from the perspective of acute versus chronic disorders. This distinction is particularly important in the study of PTSD and depression because the literature has not made this distinction, and the effects may be confounded. Investigators must address numerous questions: Who is at risk of acute disorders? Who is at risk of chronic disorders? What are the predictors of long-term and short-term recovery? Are they the same or different? How might these differences guide interventions, medications, and psychotherapy? Are preventive strategies for individuals who can anticipate trauma exposure (e.g., disaster workers, police, solders, firefighters) effective for acute disorders and/or chronic disorders?

Biological, psychological, and social interventions differ for acute and chronic disorders. For instance, treatment in the acute phase must focus first on the management of injuries. In the future, as the profession learns more about the neurobiology of trauma, pharmacological prevention of the encoding of traumatic memories and generalization of anxiety/fear responses may address the biological factors of psychological distress more specifically. In contrast, future biological treatment in chronic disorders will target the generalized fear response, "autonomously" arising memories, and comorbid disorders that inhibit recovery, such as substance abuse and depression. Similarly, psychotherapy for acute PTSD appropriately focuses on reconstruction of the traumatic events to aid cognitive processing and recall; in chronic PTSD, psychotherapy must identify memories of the traumatic event that the patient may call to mind as a symbol of present stressors and anxieties. Social interventions in the acute phase of traumatic disorders focus on establishing safety, respite, and protection from secondary traumatization; in the chronic phase, management of withdrawal and social detachment is paramount.

Future investigations should clearly distinguish acute versus chronic PTSD and depression, in particular. The lack of consideration of this dimension has led to insufficient study at both ends of the spectrum and confused hypotheses. Further research on disaster and traumatic response also is needed in rarely studied areas such as acute stress disorder; traumatic depression (see Chapter 5); and the issues of family violence, substance abuse, and the effects of compensation and community interventions after major disasters such as the Gulf War (see Chapter 6) or Hurricane Andrew (see Chapter 7). Opportunities to study the effects of single-trauma stressors, as well as multievent traumas, are important to the development of psychiatry's knowledge of the effects of trauma and disaster on individuals and communities.

ADDITIONAL SUGGESTED READINGS

American Psychiatric Association, Division of Public Affairs: Idea and Information Exchange for Disaster Response. Washington, DC, American Psychiatric Press, 1993

Austin LS (ed): Responding to Disaster. Washington, DC, American Psychiatric Press, 1992

Davidson JRT, Foa EB (eds): Posttraumatic Stress Disorder: DSM-IV and Beyond. Washington, DC, American Psychiatric Press, 1993

Hodgkinson PE, Stewart M: Coping with Catastrophe: A Handbook of Disaster Management. New York, Routledge, 1991

Nader K, Pynoss RS: School disaster: planning and initial interventions. Journal of Social Behavior and Personality 8:1–23, 1993

Raphael B: When Disaster Strikes: How Individuals and Communities Cope with Catastrophe. New York, Basic Books, 1986

Spiegel D: Dissociation: Culture, Mind and Body. Washington, DC, American Psychiatric Press, 1994

Tomb D: Posttraumatic Stress Disorder: The Psychiatric Clinics of North America. Philadelphia, PA, Saunders, 1994

Ursano RJ, McCaughey BC, Fullerton CS: Individual and Community Responses to Trauma and Disaster: The Structure of Human Chaos. London, Cambridge University Press, 1994

Wilson JP, Raphael B (eds): International Handbook of Traumatic Stress Syndromes. New York, Plenum, 1993

Index

*Page numbers printed in **bold** type refer to tables or figures.*